THE LONGEVITY REMEDY

by Sherzod Kayumov

In this book, human life is represented as the four seasons of nature (spring, summer, autumn, and winter). The author tells about the basics of a healthy lifestyle of prophylactic activities on the basis of scientific data and gives beneficial methods on how to maintain and increase the human capacity. There are so many examples in which a human can have great opportunities to extend life and decelerate aging. The book includes several helpful tips regarding the seasonal sicknesses of nature, the causes of their appearance, prevention, and treatments for them. The author hopes that the thoughts expressed in the book will help a wide population live a healthier life and fight noxious habits. At the end of the book, you can find some bonuses concerning the best way of living life.

All Secrets you want to know about Longevity are hidden in this Book!

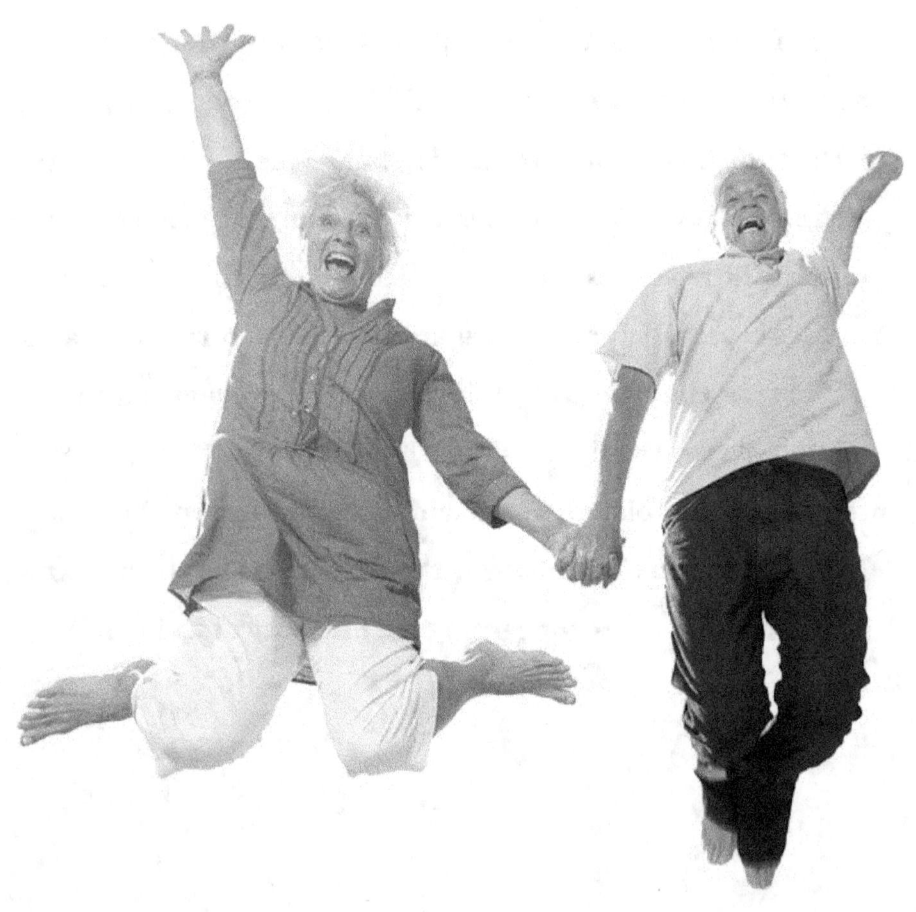

CONTENTS

Introduction

Man wants to live forever. But life is given once. Man cannot conclude that old age and death are inevitable. In this one-time life, a man dreams about living a healthy life and being young and strengthful. But could we hold the time!? Years pass by one after another. In my opinion, health is a huge wealth of human life, and the only person who perceives or appreciates this concept before he experiences trouble will not suffer a painful end. Al-Biruni says that "Human life is one hundred twenty years naturally, as the world is built up by the sun and that period is the longest year of construction". Though human can naturally live until 120 years, this is only for a lucky few with an inherited tendency to longevity.

Our body is a great self-renewing mechanism. One of the most complex tasks of modern biology is to determine the aging process of the human body and also supreme organisms, including the mechanism of death first.

Folk medicine and modern medicine cannot eliminate the aging process, even death too. The father of early modern medicine, Avicenna said:

> *"From the nadir of Earth to the zenith of Saturn,*
> *I settled all the issues of the universe.*
> *I comprehended and resolved all knotted problems,*
> *But the only remained one was the quietus."*

However, folk and modern medicine can save elderly people from a variety of old age-related diseases. The struggle to extend human life and slow down premature aging is the responsibility and noble duty of modern biology and medicine; But, it is significantly important to keep in mind that in this struggle

there is a major role of a person himself too. In order to get rid of the intrusive thoughts, it is necessary for a man to build and follow a healthy lifestyle.

The task in this area is to eliminate harmful habits, to try to avoid severe mental emotions, to develop a rational order of nutrition, environment, work and acceptable behavior in society. In doing so, it is necessary to monitor the procedure of improving the ecological situation.

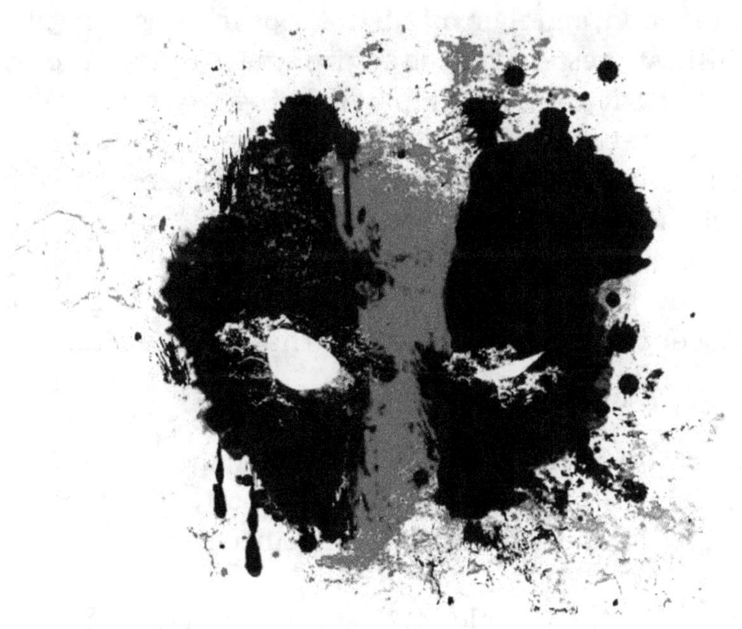

CHAPTER I

The Human Life Cycle

"I lifted all the loads, but there's not heavier load than onus, but I didn't find much more flavor than health. The most delicious flavor is health."

(Luqman)

After experiencing the phases of infancy, childhood, and youth, a human being reaches adolescence, emerging & early adulthood, and then maturity. In psychology, maturity is the ability to respond to the environment in an appropriate manner. Maturity also encompasses being aware of the correct time and place to behave and knowing when to act according to the circumstances and the culture of the society one lives in. A man reaches full maturity approximately at the age of 40. Wherefore the wise say "Man will be entirely built at the age 40". According to Avicenna, 40 years of age is the beginning of the senescence. Dante and Bacon say that the life after the age of 35 bears human to aging.

Hippocrates indicates that a limit between the old age and youth is the age 42. People who lived until 60 (Avicenna), 65 (Bacon), 63 (Hippocrates) years are specified to be old men.

Since ancient times people have been dreaming about forever being young, preserving solidarity and strength and preventing premature aging.

By doing relevant experiments with longevity issues Avicenna determines that to live a long and warm life, one significantly has to be open-minded, sweet-mouthed, genuine, open-minded and optimistic rather than be ignorant, sorrowful, voracious and smoke a cigarette or drink. He writes that "If regular exercise is being done, there is no need to use medicines."

It's written on church books that the longest-lived person was English, Thomas Kari, who was born in London and he lived for 207 years. Thereby, the limit of the human life cannot be concluded until 70-80 years but may include 100, 150, or even two centuries. By taking this objective fact into consideration, it is said that life expectancy will not be less than 150-170 years in the future.

For the first time during childhood, for the second time during late adulthood man becomes childish, the point is, at the first childish phase people caress him, at the second childish one they vainly laugh at him. If a human's nativity (just like dawn), his habitation (just like sunrise, daytime, and sunset), his aging and death (just like the red fading sun) are based on the rules of life and nature, they are closely affined to the encounter with different circumstances, incurrence upon diverse problems, surrounding environments (the air, light, water, earth), human lifestyle, his spiritual condition, and his mood.

Each person experiences a number of transition periods, depending on his age, such as marriage, pregnancy, nativity, infancy, childhood, youth, adolescence, early adulthood, climacteric period, middle adulthood and old age. There are interdependence and similarity between human lifestyle and the seasons of living nature. Based on the observations of the human life cycle, I'm going to describe the example of the 100-year-old man by contrast with four seasons of the year (spring, summer, autumn, winter) in the form of "a Mirror of Human Life". Actually, It is indefinite for human beings that how long they can survive to go through those periods.

Human life is so vast, incomparable and complexible ocean that we can not know where the beginning and the ending are.

This is clear only to the Creator.

 A human is not living in the five-day world, but living in the three-day one, that is, he was born, lived and died. Life is a struggle for a living. As we know it, we do not pay attention to the phrase "The Fight for Health". In other words, we live without noticing that harmful habits which are commonplacé in house-hold issues, while eating, clothing, working & resting, natural physiological processes in the transition periods and some un-pleasantnesses awfully damnify our health. Who wants to die early?! Human lives with dreams and hopes. But the birth, life, and death are real!

 According to the scientists, if someone does a better and reward-ing job with a good mood in a peaceful life, he will not suffer until the last point of life, he will live with happiness. Human experi-ences the natural physiological process (climacteric period) at the ages of his 40-50-60. It equalizes human's life with the end of summer and the beginning of autumn. The climacteric period is the aging stage of the human body. Could we hold the seasons, time and life?! The time and life pass fast like the wind and a flow-ing river. With his never-ending quests, uninterrupted work, the romance of the first love with his wonderful youth - the spring of human life (1-25 years) expires.

 The most productive, constructive and enterprising period of early adulthood - the summer of human life (25-50 years), vide-licet, mature years arrive. But years pass by one after another. Middle adulthood - the autumn of human life (50-75 years) also arrives. A person begins to suffer Alzheimer's disease, insomnia, excessive fatigue, and lung squeeze, vision and hearing become worse, work capacity reduces, various diseases disturb, if the weather is bad, joints start to hurt, and so on. After autumn, the stage of late adulthood (old age) -the winter of human life (75-100 years) arrives. This is the last stage of human develop-ment. Dr. Gray Bird, examining 400 people over the age of 100, concludes: "Many of these people have made a solid plan about the future, they are actively involved in the congregation work, they are energetic like young people, they have a healthy appetite, they are prone to mild jokes, life-resistant, optimistic and even the risk of death is beyond their grasp".

According to the determined data, the human organism can be reborn at the age of 90, as if the second time, even the third time rebirth may happen. The only requirement for this is that a person should live an active life. Essentially, unless the person is cold-blooded and indifferent, nothing can cool him up. These statements are supported and confirmed by our contemporaries who are in the 75's, 80's, 90's, and 100's or older. It is well known that as the person grows older he becomes more experienced and wiser, he becomes eager to share his life experience with others and try to teach his knowledge to young people.

The ancient physicians say that a person's behavior, health, and longevity depend on his sensation, emotions, and anxiety. Love, Joy, Friendship, Goodwill accompany the laughter & smile and make him more healthy and stronger.

Anxiety, anger, envy, especially fear and panic fill the mind of a person with grief shortening his life, destroying the body and breaking the heart, and then he starts to suffer from various diseases such as diarrhea, diabetes mellitus, neurosis, gastric ulcer, tuberculosis, infarction, stroke, etc.

Mental workers should never forget that their muscles, heart and blood vessels need action too. As well as persons who are engaged in physical labor or activities should not lose their interest in science, arts and artistic creation. Many people, long-lived ones, say that there are two sources of longevity.

The first is the natural resources (e.g. sunlight, water, air, earth's natural wealth, the vegetal world, etc.), climate and so forth. The second source is that we have some kind of features like We enjoy our lives, do not envy others, do not keep evil in our soul, are more cheerful and less weeping, do share joy and sorrow with others, do wake up with the sun and do sleep as the sun goes down, do love labor, do know how to relax.

Our wise people say that lazy and evil person does not live long. Thereby, everyone's health and longevity are determined by whether they do follow the correct and healthy lifestyle or not. Because, as I said before, our body is a glorious and marvelous self-renewing mechanism. Based on this enactment, in nature, animate and inanimate life prevalent and intriguing natural phenomena, as well as processes, are observed to exist. For instance, throughout the year in the macrocosm the phase conditions of the sun (such as Nowruz, summer and winter chill, etc.), the gradually and cyclically changeable moon over the period of a synodic month, starting and ending periods of days for a week (Monday and Sunday), conditions of a day (morning sunrise, evening sunset), the origin and evolution of vegetation and animal kingdom, their reproduction, senescence and so on.

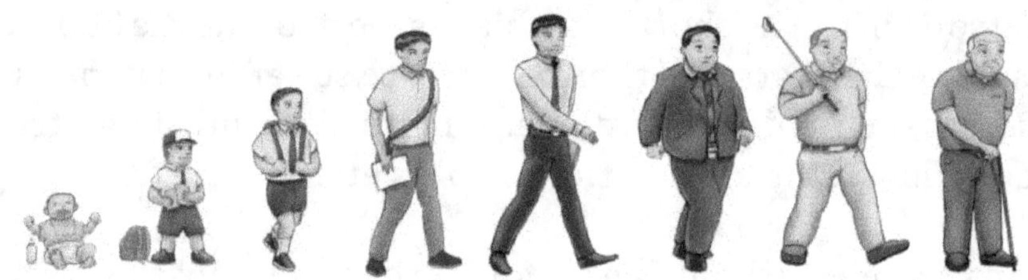

CHAPTER II

The Female Climacteric (Menopause)

The climacterium is a physiological period that the generative function of the body ceases. It is observed in both males and females.

In the climacteric period, female menstruation is changeable, and functional variations happen in the ovaries, the Pituitary (The major endocrine gland. A pea-sized body attached to the base of the brain, the pituitary is important in controlling growth and development and the functioning of the other endocrine glands), and the hypothalamus (A region of the forebrain below the thalamus that coordinates both the autonomic nervous system and the activity of the pituitary, controlling body temperature, thirst, hunger, and other homeostatic systems, and involved in sleep and emotional activity).

In males, the number of cells which produce genital hormones in testis is reduced, changes occur in the cardiovascular system, The pathological climacteric is accompanied by endocrine, vegetative and psychological changes. The climacterium is gradual suspense in female and male reproductive and sexual activities, accompanied by a general change in the body due to its growth. The climacteric is noticed in both men and women, occasionally in the youth as well. In most women, the climacteric begins at the age of 45 50, and the early climacteric begins at the age of 35-36, however, the late one may begin after old age.

Sometimes the early climacteric, which is seen in young people, is mainly caused by angina (A condition marked by severe pain in the chest, often also spreading to the shoulders, arms, and neck, caused by the inadequate blood supply to the heart), influenza (A highly contagious viral infection of the respiratory passages causing fever, severe aching, and catarrh, and often occurring in epidemics), chronic tonsillitis (We should note that there are two types of tonsillitis, to wit, acute and chronic ones. Acute tonsillitis is an infection of the tonsils caused by one of several types of bacteria or viruses. Chronic tonsillitis is a persistent infection of the tonsils and can cause tonsil stone formation.

 Signs and symptoms of tonsil or adenoid infection include a sore throat. Fever), antritis and other diseases.

 The period is observed to continue from three to five years. In some women, this period may pass smoothly. But this process is heavier for more than 30 percent of them. The climacteric may be hereditary and at the different ages too. The age at which the mother suffers the period and her daughters will suffer at the same age too. Some females don't take it seriously though there may be a risk of neurosis and adverse changes in the heart, especially in the nervous system. Many women think that the period will be passed if menstrual blood does not come up to one year. But heavy bleeding is seen to happen after a break and that testifies to the presence of various risky tumors in the genitals. So then, the medications as "Tranexamic Acid (Hemostan)" and "Dydrogesterone (Duphaston)" are prescribed to normalize hormones. According to the scientists and physicians, the period is not a disease, but the natural physiological process. The variations related to the period, mostly, disappear spontaneously, because over time the organism adapts to the new physiological circumstances. Those changes will pass faster on condition that a female follows healthy eating and lifestyle advised by the doctor. The first symptom of the period in females is principally a malfunction of the menstrual cycle.

 Some females usually experience a menstrual period once 3- 4 months, but others conversely go through this twice a month. Menstrual blood bleeds with a periodic pause, sometimes it flows lengthily and plentifully, and finally, it completely stops which is called Menopause, and ovaries' functionality deteriorates. Women who are taller, have had children and are in perimenopause have the heaviest flow.

The usual length of menstrual bleeding is four to six days. The usual amount of blood loss per period is 10 to 35 ml. Each soaked normal-sized tampon or pad holds a teaspoon (5ml) of blood.

In some women, it may be normal to have less bleeding during menstrual periods. Less blood flow may be genetic and, if inquiries are made, it may be found that a woman's mother and/or sister also have decreased blood flow during their periods. But normal problems at other times can also cause scanty blood flow. During pregnancy, pink or brown discharge or spotting before a period may be an early sign of pregnancy. This discharge is caused by implantation bleeding that can happen when the fertilized egg burrows into the uterus lining. Heavy for one woman may be normal for another. Most women will lose less than 16 teaspoons of blood (80ml) during their period, with the average being around 6 to 8 teaspoons. Heavy menstrual bleeding is defined as losing 80ml or more in each period, having periods that last longer than 7 days, or both. When a woman loses a lot of blood during her period, her iron levels can drop. This can cause anemia. She passes clots of blood and soaks through her usual pads or tampons every hour for 2 or more hours.

Nonsteroidal anti-inflammatories (NSAIDs), such as ibuprofen, or Advil can be used to treat dysmenorrhea or painful menstrual cramps, and they can help reduce blood loss. However, NSAIDs can also increase the risk of bleeding. At the female climacteric the temporary and different following symptoms may appear: a woman becomes very grumpy and moody, causelessly impatient, she loses sleep, memory, appetite and her taste changes, has a headache, her work doesn't go well and heart beats fast, she feels pain on the chest, sometimes the blood flows high in the head, her face reddens, her body burns and hurts then she becomes cold, she tires and her ears ring. If the blood in the head flows highly, she lacks strength and feels unable to work and it may require special treatment. Sometimes such kind of symptoms like emotional instability, disturbance, feeling the crabby and irritable mood, unnecessary laughing or crying and fear may appear, arterial pressure rises, dizziness, neuroticism, and psychopathic increase are seen to happen. In some cases, involutional psychosis occurs. After the end of a period, occurred changes gradually disappear and a woman feels good.

In most women, the period passes with no sharp changes and they do not feel bad. Though some women go through unpleasant sensations at that time, namely, several times a day, suddenly the blood flows in the face and neck for a short time, the skin flushes and whitens, later perspires. She gets terrified and fashed by herself, becomes jittery, sorrowful, irritable, weeping. It's called anticlimactic neurosis.

Sometimes cardiovascular function gets disordered, and a pain appears on the heart area and chest from time to time, heart beats fast or slow, arterial pressure increases, head spins, and ears ring, it feels like ants are shinning on the body.

Here are some helpful tips for females who are in the process of a climacteric period and who are stepping on it:

1. Women, after the age of 40, should definitely go to the check-ups of gynecologist twice a year and go to oncologist annually.

2. Do not forget that, during the period, severe stress of the nerves can cause serious tumors to appear in the brain.

3.   Following tips may help you if your body starts to sweat and your heart beats irregularly:

-    On a standing upright or sitting position, keep holding your hands straight over your head for 4-5 minutes;

-    Thoroughly mix a spoon of yarrow, half glass of hops, two spoons of hawthorn flowers and licorice leaves. Then take two spoons of this mixture, pour a liter of boiling water over it. Then add some honey and consume 50 g of it 3-4 times a day in warm condition and 20 minutes before the meal.

4.   It is essential to take additional hormones and micronutrients through the advice of a physician to facilitate the occurring changes to pass, maintain the general activity, prevent the enhancement of diseases, and stop the aging process.

5.   Take your regular meals at the same time every day (4 times a day, if possible). Reduce consumption of salt, meat, oil, fried foods, butter, flour, and pasta products, and consume predominantly dairy products and vegetable side dishes instead. Avoid drinking alcohol, smoking, and spices namely horseradish, mustard, peppers, sharp sauces;

6.   To maintain sexual activity, add products which are fortified with high amounts of Zn (Zinc) and Blackmores (Bio Zinc) to your rational diet;

7.   Increase whole grains (such as millet, buckwheat, quinoa, oats, rye, and barley), cruciferous vegs and, kinds of seafood, with olive oil, consume porridges made from peasemeal or cornstarch, then drink a boiled cow's milk;

8.   Eat fruits (e.g. orange, mandarin, banana, apple, grape, and other melon and watermelon).

9.   Add malted bran of rice or barley to different salads, while your meals must include cinnamon, squash, chopped pumpkin seeds, ginger, parsley, walnuts, peanuts, and almonds.

10.   It is necessary to eat soy products. Because soy reduces the intensive Hypertension (abnormally high blood pressure).

11.   You should not eat mustard, horseradish, pepper, paprika, sharp sauces, bitter tea, coffee, cocoa and so on.

12.   During climacteric, a person is inclined to get constipated. Therefore it is important to keep in mind that the digestive system is functioning properly.

13.   You should do exercises every morning and take a shower or wipe your body with water at home temperature during the day.

14.   Take a valerian bath 1-2 hours a week to protect against depression. To do this, pour 1 liter of water over 50 g of chopped valerian root, boil it for 15 minutes with low heat, leave it in a closed container for 3-4 hours and pour it into a hot water bath with a flipper.

15.   It benefits your blood if you move more and take a fresh air walk.

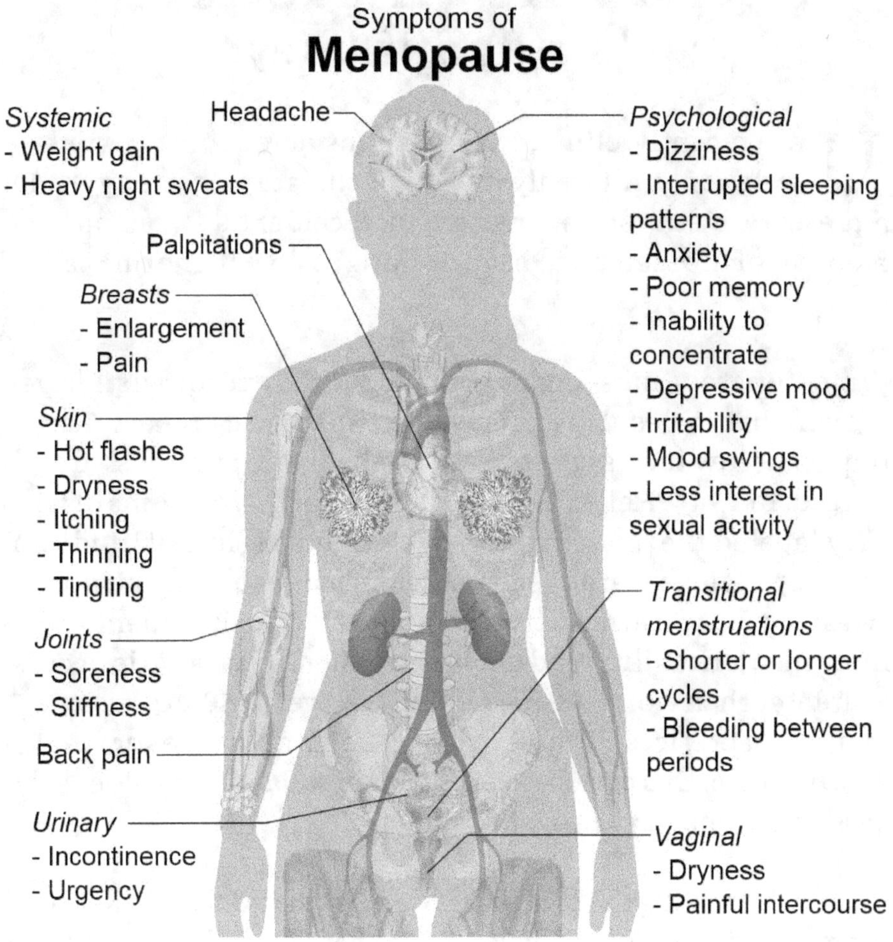

Symptoms of
Menopause
Headache
Psychological
- Dizziness
- Interrupted sleeping patterns
- Anxiety
- Poor memory
- Inability to concentrate
- Depressive mood
- Irritability
- Mood swings
- Less interest in sexual activity
Systemic
- Weight gain
- Heavy night sweats
Palpitations
Breasts
- Enlargement
- Pain
Skin
- Hot flashes
- Dryness
- Itching
- Thinning
- Tingling
Joints
- Soreness
- Stiffness
Back pain
Urinary
- Incontinence
- Urgency
Transitional menstruations
- Shorter or longer cycles
- Bleeding between periods
Vaginal
- Dryness
- Painful intercourse

CHAPTER III

The Male Climacteric (Andropause)

Until recently, climacteric was considered the issue for females only. Allegedly it was not threatening strong gender representatives. Mood swings, angina, accidental sweat, ups & downs of life seemed to have nothing to do with hormonal changes.

Unfortunately, most endocrinologists and andrologists have proven that males also experience climacteric process. The impact of low levels of testosterone has been previously reported. In 1944, Heller and Myers identified symptoms of what they labeled the "male climacteric" including loss of libido and potency, fatigue, nervousness, the inability to concentrate, sweating, hot flushes, increased body fat, impaired memory, insomnia, irritability, and depression. Men's climacteric occurs a bit later than women's one around the ages of 50-60. In some men, climacteric is variable and may begin at the ages of 30-35 or 70. Of course, this period does not begin suddenly and does not pass simultaneously in every person.

Notwithstanding the fact that it befalls everyone. Detailed and profound investigations have shown that at the ages of 50 and 60, the male egg tissue begins to alter its attribute, and the production of testosterone (One of the most active male hormones) is reduced. A high level of it drops in the blood. This hormone participates in many processes which occur in the body. All the glands in the endocrine system are interdependent. If any of these is disordered, it affects the configuration of other glands. Low testosterone is an impetus for the connection between eggs, hypothalamus and pituitary to be broken.

Consequently, it is observed that not only sexual orientation suspends but also the Secretion (A process by which substances are produced and discharged from a cell, gland, or organ for a particular function in the organism or for excretion) of prostate (A gland surrounding the neck of the bladder in male mammals and releasing prostatic fluid) and spermatoceles (A fluid-filled sac that grows in the epididymis. That's a small tube near the upper testicle that collects and transports sperm. Spermatoceles vary in size. They typically don't hurt, but they could cause pain if they grow too large) will decrease.

Further, the metabolism is broken, and the tonus of the muscles and skin tissues decreases. There are huge differences between the physiologic and pathologic climacterics. The unpleasant phenomenon can be caused by physiology, i.e., naturally (related to aging), and also pathology, as a result of various diseases (which is why male climacteric may start early). The only difference is that in the first instance, the organism is able to adapt to new conditions and live in harmony with change. The second instance is quicker and harder. In physiological climacteric, a person is often tired, has a tendency to mental suffering (depression), changes in bone structure, tissue destruction, anemia, osteoporosis, obesity, memory loss, frequent drowsiness, hypertension, increased sweating, pulse-rate acceleration, dizziness, migraine, and abdominal bloating are observed to happen. Aging process and aggravating conditions (such as diabetes mellitus, ischemic heart disease, blood pressure, smoking, alcohol abuse, etc.) may deepen the above symptoms. Pathological climacteric is accompanied by changes in mentality, cardiovascular system, urinary system, and vascular system disorders. It is said that sudden or severe colds or fever, rapid rise or fall in blood pressure, and obesity may occur. Patients complain about the high incidence of insomnia and excitability. A person who experiences the periodic symptoms will often have difficulty to understand it.

Here are some beneficial tips for males who are in the process of a climacteric period and stepping on it:

1. As soon as you live an active lifestyle and do not drink alcohol and smoke less, you will not need to be afraid of the adventurous signs of andropause, that is to say, climacteric passes quickly and unnoticeably.

2. If you are highly likely to do telecommuting, if you are not sports-friendly, if you like to spend time with a cup of beer in the sofa, you should take a break after the age of 40 and start to live an active healthy lifestyle.

3. Those who are engaged in physical training need to continue it, and those who are not have to start with morning exercise and hiking.

4. Your health depends on the harmony in family relationships, so keep on giving gifts to your spouse, do not neglect her, take interest in upbringing, education, and works of your children and care for them.

5. Do not overwork and exceed 8 hours. Most importantly, never leave any problems outside of your office.

6. Do not allow long-term nervous and physical stress.

7. Always dress depending on the weather and get neither hot nor cold.

8. Put the composition of food in such a way that the high quantity of fat should be reduced, and increase proteins, micro-nutrients, minerals, and vitamins. Limit fried foods.

9. Live in an Active Sex Life. Only then you will not be disturbed by genital aging. In my opinion, it wouldn't be wrong if men accepted natural support.

10. According to scientists, unfortunately, pathological climacteric cannot be prevented. Sometimes doctors also cannot tell why hormonal changes are occurring earlier. Therefore, if you notice the symptoms of climacteric, seek medical advice immediately.

11. As far as possible, describe the doctor about the things that cause you disturbing, and ask to carry out the following checks:

  - Determine the level of testosterone in the blood;

  - Dopplerography of reproductive organs;

  - Diagnosis of prostate-specific antigen.

12.   In some cases, light hormonal therapy is performed. This method of treatment can be used when excessive physiological climacteric disturbs. Therefore, we, men, need to pay attention to our women as much as possible in the climacteric period to help our women not lose confidence in themselves. Because trust in themselves is beneficial not only for them but for family, for children, for relatives, for those around and also for our community. Climacteric must not lead to a change in the harmonious marriage of the couple. But in this period, the husband should concern his wife and the wife should do the same to her husband with special care and attention and help each other to experience the most difficult time in life. Generally, it is essential to raise our women, one of the marvels of nature, to the sky and embosom them tightly.

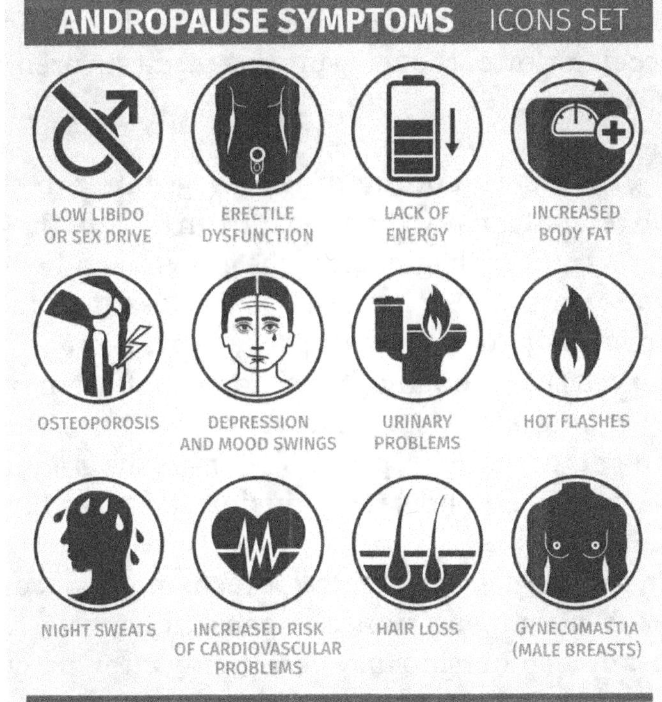

CHAPTER IV

Is Old Age Pleasure or Affliction?

Old age is the last stage of human development. Old age, aging is a legitimate process as a result of variations occurring in the body by deterioration with age. These variations gradually lead the adaptability of an organism to life to decline.

Aging is the appearance of "fatigue" in some organs and tissues, as well as in the whole body. Aging is the end of the individual development of an organism, which is considered conditional on the person starting at the age of 75. This is physiologic aging. When physiologic aging begins, mental and physical power, particular workability, cheerfulness and interest in the environment are preserved. Due to the varied adverse effects and internal factors, acceleration of the aging process results in premature or pathological aging.

Typically, the first symptoms of aging begin after the age of adulthood (conditionally the age of 60). In spite of the fact that the aging process begins after the growth and development of the organism. For instance, at the ages of 30 and 35, the level of activity of biological processes is decreasing. It has been observed that the aging process does not begin simultaneously in different tissues and organs, vice versa there are different levels of the aging process. Aging is the gradual cessation and loss of a cell's power of division and growth.

However, due to the physiological, biochemical and other mechanisms of compensation, compensation for the full or partial loss of membership may be felt only after many of its cells have been disengaged. This type of compensation is largely dependent on the body's adaptability which is developed during the active life cycle. However, while growing older, in preserved cells the activity of the oxidation process gradually begins to fade away, oxygen consumption in tissues decreases, the eyes become blurred, the ears do not hear well, the endurance of respiratory capacity and muscle strengths drops piecemeal, but mostly it cannot be perceived for a long time when doing normal and less painful work.

The changes initially initiated by aging, however, practically do not break the adaptability of the body's acute changes in life, but with increasingly gradual aging and changes, the organism becomes more adaptable to these changes.

Particularly, it is known during physical and mental stresses. The aging process primarily affects the cardiovascular and nervous systems.

The cardiovascular system provides cells, tissues, and organs with a full range of specific tension during the aging process. It, in turn, is the process of decomposition. In elderly people, due to the deterioration of the mobility of the nervous system, it is difficult to initiate and work. Insufficient braking is accompanied by an increase in excitation of the nervous system, therefore, conditional reflexes, which are the basis of adaptation to the response reactions and surrounding objects, passively work and then fade away and emotional instability increases.

Aging is often accompanied by various chronic illnesses, which can lead to premature aging. In general, there is a certain correlation between age-specific changes and illness. In the process of aging, the body's abilities to gain flexibility and recovery may retard that leads to the development of diseases and the more severe transition of them. Therefore, preventing the disease will help prevent premature aging.

There is no single idea about the causes of aging currently, but the theory that aging depends on the genetic apparatus of the cells is widespread. Hence, genetics can be regarded as momentous in the aging process. Attention has long been given to the extended long-living people in some families.

Hereditary features in such families are observable through their slow aging and disease-resistance.

There are many problems in the world. However, in many's best interests, there may not be a great problem as aging. The death is real, therefore, it is natural that everybody is interested in knowing how many hours left to live their lives. In addition to the theory that the aging process is related to the genetic apparatus, researches by the world scientists have shown that aging can be led by a variety of factors. For instance, academician V. Engelgardt (Russia) says that "Certainly, as the life of any living being, human life is also limited. But it is not clear what kind of limitation it is, and today we do not know if we have reached this boundary or not. For this reason, the usage of "opportunities" such as lowering the risk of child mortality and fighting dangerous diseases has not yet been substantiated. Thus social factors play a crucial role in resolving this issue. The development of enzymology revealed that the change in the properties of biological catalysts controlling all processes of metabolism in the body is the most important factor in aging processes. Recently, the important biological role of cell and other membranes has become evident. Mayhap the changes in membrane properties lead to aging".

The famous Australian biologist M. Burnet, a developer of modern immunological theory, says that "The longevity is associated more by satisfaction and moral behavior than by the factors of physical exercise, hiking, long-lived parents, avoiding alcohols and smoking. Obviously, an amazing internal defense mechanism called the Immune System protects the body from bacteria and viruses that can lead to illness. A healthy immune system produces a variety of different cells to attack the Foreign Invaders entering the body, and possibly involves the destruction of mutants, that is, abnormal cells. The most important part of the immune system, in my opinion, is the thyroid gland. Probably, it produces the lymphocytes which normalize the immune response. The actual lymphocytes themselves find foreign cells and connect with them and eat them.

Shortly after childbirth, the production of lymphocytes in the gland greatly accelerates while the thyroid becomes enlarged. When the child reaches the age of 10-12, the thyroid extremely enlarges and then slowly shrinks. In most people over the age of 60, only two pieces of fibrous tumor tissue located at the thyroid remain. This does not mean that lymphocytes will disappear in elderly people. It contains many remnants of cells that once produced glands, but no new cells appear. Perhaps, as human goes to the end of his life many cells in the body can be transformed into abnormal cells. Therefore, some scientists believe that aging is a consequence of just a collection of mutations. Other scientists (including myself) have different views on this issue.

My attitude to the issue of aging is that although mutations can play an important role in the process, the reduction of the immune system will also have a significant impact on the aging process. The main appearance of aging is the vulnerability. The older people are more susceptible to influenza, bronchitis, bronchopneumonia and the like. This is the first indication that the organism's ability to disinfect the disease rapidly fades away. Being diagnosed with cancer in old age is due to the two main causes - the accumulation of abnormal cells and the suspense of the "immunological control" which destroys cancer when it begins to appear.

Moreover, in many people, old age begins with many diseases. When a person becomes very weak, he dies of various and sometimes random phenomena too".

Usually, an aged person is imagined to be weak and have thin-wrinkled skin. These exterior features are mainly due to the lack of the so-called collagen substance, which provides for the extracorporeal protein, the strength, and elasticity of the connective tissue. Collagen is the most important substance that boosts the body, improves bone resistance.

Collagen deficiency is manifested in people over 70 years. As we grow older, not only thyroid but also all the lymphoid tissues-the spleen, the lymphatic glands, the marrow, and the others gradually shrink. But the thyroid regenerates more quickly than the rest. After 40 or 50 years of age, the thyroid will not work almost immediately. And in the old age, this gland completely disappears.

Given the above, we consider that the loss of the thyroid is currently the most appropriate factor in the interpretation of aging. Perhaps it is possible to say that "Biological clock" can be found in the thyroid and related cells. When the "Simple repair" of the body stops, all the illnesses that can be seen in old age will put forth.

Leonard Hayflick, a professor of Anatomy at the UCSF School of Medicine in San Francisco, discovered that tissue cells from lab-grown human meat can be separated into approximately fifty times in the most favorable conditions.

Then the division stops, and the cells die. So, apparently, there is a certain limit of the division of cells in the human body (id est 50). Hayflick is convinced that this rare occurrence was the basis of old age, and his idea was very intriguing to me. Since it gives the scope of a clear expression respecting the theories of aging.

The concept of Hayflick was about the same: every biological species has its own "biological clock", videlicet "Hayflick limit/phenomenon" - the limit of the number of divisions that can occur in the body's cells. Hence, if some vital cell lines for longevity finish "the norm of self-division" faster than the other cell lines, the age-related changes begin due to the absence of that cell.

As we know that the thyroid glands produce the lymphocytes, and the cells, originated by the lymphocytes, are separated faster than the other cells. Fibroblasts which controls the formation of collagen may finish its own period early.

Besides, they are made up of the specialized cell which forms immune cells. If it is true, then all these cells at the same time, that is to say, before the actuation, the rest of the body will reach the "Hayflick limit" earlier. And it means the beginning of aging.

Doctor of Biological Sciences A.Neyfakh puts forward M.Barnette's theory and other issues that are important for understanding the aging.

- The essence of Barnette's theory is, Neyfakh says, at first the thyroid gland "gets old" in the human body. The reason is that the thyroid gland cells can divide until 50 as Hayflick said. Thereafter, the efficiency of defensive activity of lymphocytes is reduced. Some of the abnormal cells become cancer cells, and the rest cause other disorders. As a result, they lead to senescence. Barnette believes that cancer is the consequence of a naturally or artificially created changes (mutation) of an organism's genetic features that cannot be stood by an organism's immune system for some reason.

Indeed, there is much information about mutations which lead to the poorer quality variation of cells. However, the issue of the origin of cancer is more complicated than mutations. In this process, an oncogene (tumor-generating virus genes, capable of promoting the growth of dangerous cells) and oncogenic substances which are capable of tumor enhancement (Carcinogen) play an important role.

The issue of "foreign proteins" that develops on the tumor is also quite complex. Barnette says cancer cells form foreign proteins. Nongranular white blood cell -one of the types of leukocyte (lymphocyte), determines the proteins and then produces antibodies against them. Is this idea true?

The famous immunologist G.Abelev achieved to find separate proteins that are formed in some tumor cells and excreted to the blood. He developed the immunological method of early detection of certain types of cancer on the basis of such proteins. However, these specific proteins of tumors are not alien, and they appear in a healthy body even during the development of an embryo. Therefore, the lymphocytes consider them "theirs" and do not produce antibodies against them. How do these arguments fit Barnette's theory? How can the cancer of the thyroid that occurs in young people and even in children be explained by the Barnett theory? Perhaps at this time the types that form the "self-proteins" of the same tumors originate, and because of the resistance of the thyroid gland, tumor types that form foreign proteins can appear?! Such suppositions come close to the fact.

I would like to highlight another issue that is important in understanding the problems of aging. What is the role of genetic and environmental factors in this regard?

For example, let's take a look at the psychic image of a person such as the mental capacity, the social status, and so on.

Obviously, much of this is defined from the childbirth to one's upbringing, education, developmental conditions, environment, and perhaps the occurrence of random events in life. However, the genetic ability inherited by ancestors plays an important role in the formation of one's personality. Seemingly, life expectancy depends on external condition too. Even if wars or similar accidents are not counted, lifetime will change depending on the type of nutrition, smoking, alcohol consumption, and various ailments. The genetic identification of the main feature of aging is a primary task, and we still know little about it. Undoubtedly, the subsequent complex research shows the role of the immune system in the process of aging and the relation of Barnette's interesting theory. Many scientists believe that aging is due to the intensive division of body cells and the decrease in the ability of self-renewal of tissues. As the age grows older, the protein exchange in the body also breaks down. There is also a reduction in fat exchange: the subcutaneous fat increases and it accumulates more in the tissue too. The inadequacy of water in the body results in wrinkles. The composition of the bones also changes and bones become finer and thinner. The mobility of the spine and synovia between joints decreases, the walking style, and figure change, and height lowers.

Aging is not only the cessation of the developmental process but also the development of new conditions that support natural processes in the body. The genetic factor is of great importance herein. That is dependent on the longevity of long-lived people's children and their close relatives.

It is known that in the lifespan not only the effect of the genetic factor is significant but the effect of the external environment as well. That's why an aging person should be able to accurately assess his or her body's abilities, and keep himself safe from physical and psychological tension. Aging primarily affects the cardiovascular and nervous system.

Normal nutritional suppression prevents obesity, ergo "atherosclerosis", blood pressure, diabetes, joints, and chronic diseases too. Due to the reduction of exchange processes, the body feels less need for food. Therefore, consuming less animal fat, sugar, bread, potatoes, and porridges are recommended.

Also, to prevent digestive tract and chronic liver, kidney diseases, it is reasonable to avoid bitter, salty, sweet, oily, very hot or cold foods and appetizers. The first reason for the premature aging is the muscular inactivity. Muscle movements are the body's necessity. Therefore, no matter what the person is engaged in, certain exercises are needed throughout his life. For the sake of the elderly, morning exercise is of great importance. Simultaneously at a specified time, daily tours in nature are the most healthy important moments in the life of everyone.

As with all the members and systems in the body, it is the harmonization of work and relaxation for the cells that form them. During the relaxation period, the large cell collects materials for itself and uses them during the work. Due to the constant exchange of strict rhythm as well as work and pleasure, the members of our bodies work hard for the rest of life. Broken rhythm and immersing into the work can lead to chronic fatigue. And, conversely, adapting the passive relaxation is a risk for members to become inactive. Thus, in both cases, the organism gets sick because of a malfunction and the life span decreases. Thereupon, there should be the rhythm in all aspects of life since childhood.

It is important to emphasize that sexual life has a great impact on the prolongation of healthy and harmonious life. Apparently, the activity of the genital glands has a strong effect on the mood of a person, even though many scientists have found that the cause of aging is the termination of the activity of the same glands.

Though one of the causes of aging related only to these glands is rare, anyway it is impossible to deny the effects of genital glands on the whole body, life span, and life rhythm. For my argument, it is enough to say that the majority of great people whose creativity hasn't been lost yet and who are spiritually mature also retained their sexual abilities even they are elderly.

The child is from the beginning, as people say, from childhood it has to be followed that the ability of the organism is infinite, therefore, misspending it can inevitably lead to a loss of ability, or even a total loss.

It should not be avoided, however, that when the body is younger, intensive sexual intercourse can have a devastating effect on the individual, but this is not the case in young people since the braking system of the brain is yet slow at a young age.

Struggle for longevity is the prevention and treatment of diseases. The correct attitude with the external environment, that is, climate, nutrition, disease-spreading microbes, and genetics have a great influence on a person's life and his health. Not just that, the social environment plays a more important role in everyone's life. Apart from external factors, it is important that a person himself should care about his behavior, character, mood, habits, and health too.

The slower flow of the aging process in women is attributed to the features of the genetic apparatus. It is likely that the slower aging of women than men also depends on other factors (for example, women are less likely to smoke or drink alcohol). In women, vascular atherosclerosis occurs later.

The malfunctional blood supply to the brain and heart is less observable in women and so forth.

Aging is characterized by a change in physical state, as well as a certain degree of mental illness, first of all, psychological distress, often mood disorder, aggravation of behavior, etc.

The occurrence and aggravation of person's age-specific changes are often known after retirement. Here some people take the old age quickly and say that "I spent all my power, and now others have to work and care for us". This misconception often leads to feelings of loneliness. Usually, reducing the activity in the old age decreases the likelihood of being together with people. Additionally, the old man is irritable and does not take a critical look at himself. Often he overvalues his opportunities and past works, thus, to him, it seems like all good things have passed through, and are now inappreciable.

Knowing the old man's mental hygiene and doing so would be to maintain a proper relationship with a family of elderly people, one of the basic conditions for an elderly person to live comfortably - to work hard, to care for people, to live among relatives, it is a feeling of the advantage. Inactivity reduces the tone of life, leads to physical weakness, and loneliness leads to distress, hopelessness, and barbarity.

Older people put big demands on people around them, especially the relatives of them. They should remember to the elderly about being kind and patient, the old man's uncertainty, the fear of the future and self-importance. When a person is old, he needs to regularly check his health to the doctor. People should act according to the change of old people's mood, in case an elderly person is disturbed and depressed, he should promptly go to a physician for the checkups.

Probably the tempo of aging varies in people, in some of them at the ages of 75 and 80, and even later, there will be strength and opportunity to engage in various activities. Nonetheless, in old age, all people have less capacity, and they get tired of doing heavy work. So even if the condition is good, it is important not to work strenuously. However, labor enthusiasm is of particular importance in factors affecting the person. Let's say it is in vain to search for a long-lived idler at the history of humanity.

Conversely, all those who have lived long lives are those who have been attached to the labor and have kept the labor enthusiasm and capacity until the end of their lives. Literally, a person's labor activity is a naturally vital condition of his life. Without labor, the organism can not have the required stimulus for its vital activity. Effective labor receives an advantage. Because the labor goes with positive emotions, it improves metabolism, activates the function of the nervous system, and so on. This has a good effect on the work of the internal organs.

Additionally, any kind of labor is bactericidal for the body and a peculiar exercise that resists the tissues and organs being languished. Observing the procedure of work and rest allows all the systems of the body to function very well. When the procedure is important, optimal rhythm is produced in the body, and that is called biological activity, ie the rhythm of changing the state of the body's work from time to time.

This kind of rhythm is overriding to the aging body, due to the fact that the body is preserved well and can do a lot of work. The right queue for work and relaxation is closely related to sleep, and sleep deprivation is more common in the elderly. Long-term disturbed sleep gradually affects the nervous system, which in turn influences the internal organs, the functioning of the cardiovascular system, and so on. It should be noted that, however, as the age grows, the need for sleep will be reduced. If the condition is worsened and extenuation is felt due to insomnia, it is necessary to get a doctor. Because of the variety of sleep deprivation, sleeping pills should be avoided or consulted with a physician. Many scientists in the world are recognizing that physical and mental indolence is a powerful factor that can shorten the human life span. For a harmonious and perfect life, it is important to combine factors such as working capacity and satisfaction.

All of the great men have been motivated to work and have shown love for their labor. There is nothing to accomplish in life without these two attributes. Pushkin, Tolstoy, Tchaikovsky, all the great men on earth have still been admired by many people because of their hard work and labor satisfaction. Even in the most difficult conditions, they worked with high quality. It should be noted that the stronger these characters in the person, the more he leaves his mark. A person should be able to feel the benefits and purpose of his labor. Purposeless labor becomes pain and suffering for a person. There might not be more punishment for him than a forced or purposeless work.

On the contrary, it turns out that the work aimed at improving the welfare of people opens the heart of a person and makes him enjoy life. For example, recall the academician I.Pavlov. He could become a spiritually young and an internally beautiful man until the end of his life. At the age of 86, he was able to keep his physical and mental strength. Only for a random reason, he died of incurable acute pneumonia at that time.

Obviously, people usually retire when they feel fatigue. This factor sometimes causes a sharp change in the habit of working, causing a feeling of loneliness that crushes the heart and a person begins to feel redundant. In most cases, the same thing happens when the administrative staff reaches the age of retirement, that is, he will be retired without the consent of, or in opposition to, his will.

This can be a tragedy for a retired person. Only those with a strong will can withstand such a crisis in life. That is why pensioners should work on their own, as it is difficult to get away from society and to break the lifestyle that is commonly used, and unfortunately, it leads to the acceleration of the aging processes.

Doing neither mental nor physical work or wasting a day by

idleness is unhealthy.

"Doing nothing is an unfortunateness of the elderly" written by 83-year-old Victor Hugo.

Scientists believe that by comparing the lives and deaths of different people, the whole life, behavior, and even aging of a person are determined by his intelligence, i.e., the central nervous system. When the human brain is highly developed, the processes inside the body are so perfect that the nature of the body is kept so long. If no particular cause breaks the balance of human, he will live long enough keeping his humanistic appearance literally until the last minute of his life.

Most scientists say that as the function of the central nervous system increases, the body's ability to interact with the surrounding environment increases and its age extends. Scientists have concluded that the correlation between brain development and life span is the comparison of a correlation between the body's age and the brain's weight.

This can be explained in the following way: the age-related changes in the central nervous system are one of the important factors of the organism's aging, that is, aging of the nervous system can lead the whole body to age. A human with a large brain usually maintains the body's vital activity even when he has grown up.

In alcoholics and chain-smokers, neurons are quickly eroded due to alcohol and tobacco. As the age grows on, the number of nerve cells decreases, then it will be insufficient to manage the organism's function, and they die prematurely.

Alcohol and tobacco shorten a person's life, not only because of its toxic effect but also by making a person wally, losing his memory, reducing his critical thinking.

Thereby, if a person has a considerably undeveloped mind, on top of that if various external or internal factors negatively impact on him, in such person the brain and the central nervous system will soon become too weak, the function of all organs and tissues is sharply reduced.

Such a person will become a lackadaisical old man even when his peers are still discerning and energetic in their life.

I. Pavlov said, "There is great power in concentration". The great inventions and discoveries of many scientists have been created as a fruit of many years of effective thinking thanks to their concentration.

Do not busy your memory on any minor unnecessary facts and figures, had better keep pocket-book, it saves your precious time, and make it easier to find the right info when needed. Sometimes it allows remembering the smallest details that are vital.

Elderly people, or especially those who engage in intellectual and creative work, are highly likely to lose their memory, and they become forgetful of many things. Well, how can this be forestalled?

THE FIRST METHOD. Relearning forgotten words in memory. The essence of this method is that a certain region of the brain associated with memory is not occupied throughout human life, it can always be used to recall forgotten words or memorize new ones.

THE SECOND METHOD. Writing household chores and service assignments down in special diary (pocket-book), marking those that are done. It should always be carried by the side and recorded on time and recording the work done several times a day.

THE THIRD METHOD. Systematically storing all items, documents, and materials in a clearly defined location. In doing so, it is easy to find what you need. Adjustment of nutrition is crucial when it comes to aging. For example, eating too much calorie foods is likely to significantly aggravate the aging process. While being inactive, eating too much food is a health hazard. In people aged 60 and over, the process of metabolism will be slightly reduced. A person should consume food little by little and variously. Food should contain protein, fat, carbohydrates, vitamins and minerals.

 The ingredients with high cholesterol (egg, brain, liver, butter, etc.) and hardly soluble oil (sheep fat, etc.) should be consumed sparingly or never be added to food. An essential amount of animal proteins and fats can be taken to account for more dairy products. Vegetables and fruit should be eaten before the meal. It is recommended to consume roasted, pickled, smoked and dried foods and limit the amount of salt. Elderly people should avoid any kind of food which multiplies sputum, as well as sharp and bitter things namely appetizers and medicines. But these can be used for treatment. It is important to be careful not to eat somniferous, analgesic and sedative drugs in the old age as well as not to drink too much-beaten coffee and bitter tea named as stimulants which affect the functioning of the nervous system. In the old age, "Bath Treatment" is essential, it stimulates the organism's flexibility and improves its resistance to diseases. However, it is important to consult a physician to know the type of them and how much time needed to engage. Because, age-related changes in the body, as well as any chronic diseases, limit the ability to use such kind of treatments and even some of them can never be used fairly.

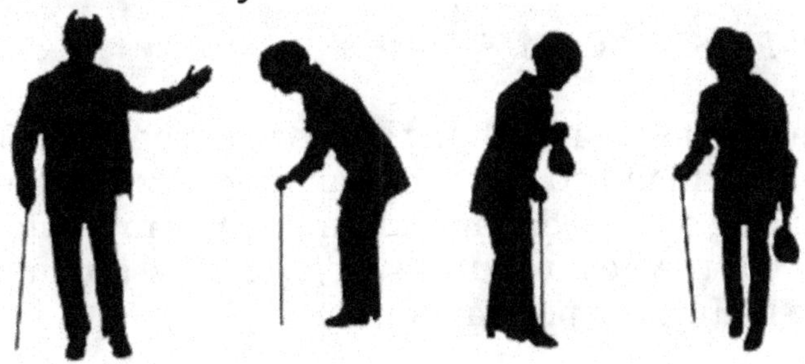

CHAPTER V

Secrets behind Longevity

Humanity has been looking for an answer to a single mystery which has tortured for a long time: How can a person live longer?

According to human heredity, 120 years of life is guaranteed. The longest-living population is estimated to be Japanese currently and the average life expectancy is 79 years, while the Australians, Greeks, Canadians, and Swedes live on average 78 years.

In the middle of the 7th century, a well-known Chinese physician Sun Simiao developed the Health and Longevity formulas. He advised as "Do not listen to a loud sound, Do not say unwanted words, Do not keep ridiculous ideas in your head and Do not overdo."

Sun Simiao said "Life is given to us to enjoy it if so it's not worth the extra tension! You do not have to worry about every simple incident. With this, I'm not just going to say sing and celebrate. Everything is good in its place. The real meaning of the word "LIFE" is "action without action" in Chinese! So be sure to change your business activity and movement state neatly! ".

HOW CAN THIS BE ACCOMPLISHED?

The ancient Chinese say "Sitting long harms the body. Sleeping long makes it difficult to breathe. Standing long damages the bones. Walking on long distances complicates muscular work." A person needs to know when to stop, rest, slow down the action and how to maintain a permanent rhythm.

The XI century scientist Xuan Tinzyan advises: "Have some rest after consuming your meal and tea. Have some rest again after daytime concerns. If you keep away from envies and heartbreaks, relaxation will bring you more bliss."

In ancient times, the wise in China showed that there is a connection between the seasons of nature and the human lifestyle, and they studied human's life by dividing into four ways. They tell everyone to be kind and healthy. They emphasized 15 suggestions for long-term survival: "Massage your face more. Hair should be constantly combed. The eyes should act steadily. Have an ear to the ground. The teeth in the upper and the lower rows need to touch each other. Close the mouth all the time. Always have saliva in the mouth.

Learn how to breathe deeply and softly. Keep your heart calm. Act consciously. Keep your shoulder straight. Rub your abdomen a lot. Make your breast stronger. Speak shortly and fluently. Let the skin have regular moisture."

In short, it is permissible for a person to be able to manage himself and know his abilities and opportunities. Accordingly, "The secret to longevity is to live properly!" such an idea comes then, does not it? Look at the lives of our ancestors.

They spoke honestly, worked industriously and ate rationally, more importantly, they lived modestly. All of this is the way to live longer as we wished. An international group of contemporary scientists, psychologists, dietologists, and doctors has developed six useful guidelines that can make the elderly enjoy a long and pleasant life. The followings are some of the factors that can extend life:

1. Do NOT eat to the FULL.

Do not exceed your eating time by 20 minutes. If you finish in 5-10 minutes, your food sits in the stomach like a heavy stone and then it difficult for it to be "discharged".

Masticate every bite 8-10 times. As a result, together with saliva, ptyalin (salubrious substance) is produced. This substance causes the stomach to work with full energy, and satiety occurs.

Do not go to bed immediately after lunch. If you are busy with some kind of affair, you will not experience gastritis, colitis, ulcers, and other gastrointestinal diseases.

Food should fit your age. Since people of all ages eat differently. 30-year-old people should consume liver and nuts while beta carotene (carrot) is optimal for 40-year-old people. After 50 years calcium keeps bone whilst magnesium benefits heart. Selenium-rich foods like cheese and kidneys are very necessary for people aged over 40. After 50 years of age, we protect our heart and blood vessels with the consumption of fish.

2. SLEEP in a COOL room.

Those who slept in a room with a temperature of 17-18 degrees will remain young for many years. Because the metabolism of the body, especially, an attribute of age depends on the environment in many respects.

3. Always BE in MOTION.

Physical training is stronger than any medication. The 8 to 10-minute morning exercise also prolongs life. For health, exercise is equalized with food and water. Thanks to the correct set of activities, it is possible to maintain the mobility of the joints until the oldest age.

It is known that the activity strengthens muscles and joints. So, engage yourself in the daytime activities immediately after you wake up.

4. Show AFFECTION, LOVE, and KINDNESS.

Love leads to the production of complex chemical substances in the body, and these substances, in turn, excite the heart. In the stomach, pleasant and warm sensations occur, and palms sweat. Thrilled people look 10 to 15 years younger. During a conversation, the body produces endorphins (happiness hormone) which strengthen the immune system.

5. MASSAGE.

This is hygienic treatment. By applying different methods of massage, you activate the protective powers of the body and feel free of emotions. As a result, the ability to work increases, mood improves, premature aging is prevented.

6. Feel SECURE and do GOOD to the PEOPLE.

Avoid psychological collisions as far as you can. Clearly, all illnesses result from nervousness. With nervous insomnia, infusions of mint, the lemon balm (melissa) and valerianne leaves are expedient. Rub your body every day with a towel that has cold salty water. Try to follow the following tips at your home and work in a mutual relationship: First, consider your collocutor's dignity, do not be angry and keep silent for a moment. Sometimes it is necessary to listen to the leader's point of view and to be humble most of the times, do not flatter your ego, kill it instead. If you look critically at yourself, you will gain the respect of others around you.

Never be alone with your concerns and disappointments. If you share them with rationalist or righteous person, you will be relieved. Treat your collocutor genuinely and heartfeltly.

Make sure your face is open during a conversation. Know your collocutor's name, and always listen to him. Let him speak about himself, then talk about in this theme. Do it in a way that his

Sherzod Kayumov

ideas are important to you, and give him a real sense of honor.

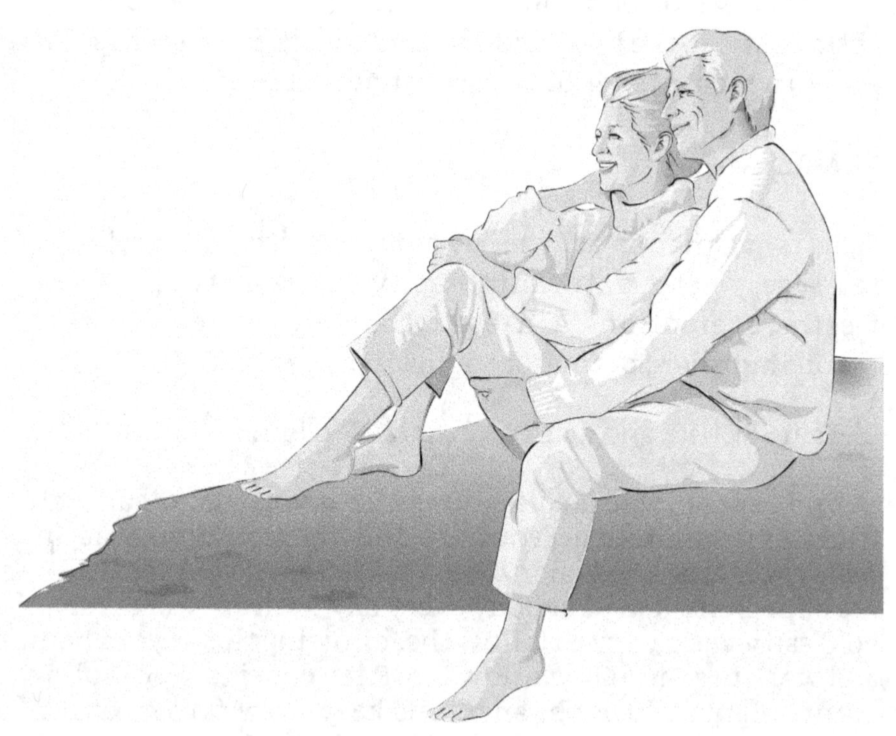

CHAPTER VI

The Treatments of Fatigue

Fatigue or strengthlessness is based on the loss of the body's previously existing capacity. It causes a number of illnesses such as malnutrition, scarcity of essential nutrients needed for tissue feeding on the body that can aggravate fatigue. In this case, it is desirable to use certain medical treatments with folk medicine, in addition to medicine.

Here are some of them:

1. First of all, take a look at your lifestyle, make some adjustments if possible: pay attention to your food, and engage in physical training. Wiping the body with a woolen tissue soaked into olive oil also results in better benefits.

Eat more roasted chickens, goose meat, porridge, nuts, honey or fructose.

2. In order to prolong life and eliminate extenuation, mix garlic with millet and heated oil, and preserve for three weeks, then consume within 21 days.

3. To prevent disease and prolong life, mix a tablespoon of chili pepper with half a kilo of oil and 200 grams of honey, it should be consumed 4-5 tablespoons a day until the mixture is ready. If needed, spend at least three months and then continue the procedure.

4. In order for the patient to recover, it is necessary to place a few pieces of freshly peeled garlic near his pillow.

5. It is recommended to eat raisins, nuts, cheeses daily and pike fish bi-weekly, in the event of chronic fatigue or after severe disease.

6.   To strengthen the whole body and increase its durability, it is necessary to drink the infusion of rose hip. To do this, put a tablespoon of rose hip into a half-liter thermos, pour boiling water, infuse it overnight, and ladle it in the morn. Drink it from half a cup three times a day and 20 minutes before a meal.

7.   The following mixture is recommended as a means of relieving the body: 350 g of red wine, 150 g of aloe vera water, 250 g of mead are added to each other. The plant should not be watered for three days before cutting the leaves off (it must be 3-5 years old). Cut leaves, then wash, chop and squeeze its water out. Mix all the ingredients and leave the prepared compound in a dark place at 4-8 degrees Celsius for a week. Consume one tablespoon of it three times a day and half an hour before a meal.

8.   Again, as a means of relieving the body, it should be thoroughly pounded by mixing a cup of raisins, two lemons, a cup of kernels of nut, and a cup of dried apricots. Pour 1.5 liters of mead, and then mix it all. Eat one tablespoon of it three times daily and an hour before a meal. For children, a teaspoon is enough.

9.   Honey has the ability to improve the overall condition of the weakened and emaciated individuals and increase the hemoglobin levels in the blood. Therefore, consuming 100-150 grams of honey every day is beneficial.

10.   Once a month, pour a decoction of thymes over yourself to strengthen the entire body and increase resistance to illness.

Below you can observe the natural remedies offered by folk medicine for the elderly:

I.   Means for regulating the function of the gastrointestinal tract:

1. Tibetan medicine recommends the following:

"You started your life with milk and porridge, finish it so".

Everyone over the age of 40 must eat at least a few spoons of porridge per day. It is a boon to the stomach, intestines, bones, and muscles.

2.   Salted cabbage juice is used as a means of strengthening the body and stomach.

3.   The watermelon which is the perfect remedy for improving the function of intestines, removing excess body waste and urine and healing kidneys is recommended to eat it once in a while.

4.   An enema should be done at least once a week in old age. Although the stomach does not bother, it is clear that long-term waste accumulates in the intestines at this age. As a result, the body is poisoned. Thus, It is helpful to drink a decoction of peppermint, mayweed, and wormwood on an empty stomach.

5.   Legume is a good body relaxer and cleaner, an effective diarrhea treater and flatulence preventer. In the old age, consuming 150-200 grams of porridge made from legume flour daily is recommended.

6.   A decoction of strawberry boosts the function of the gastrointestinal tract, opens the appetite, relaxes the viscera, increases hemoglobin level in the blood.

II.   Means for the elimination of panting and moderation of cardiovascular system and brain function:

1. Drinking a quarter cup of milk every day stops panting.

2. Drinking bitter tea is the best way to stop bleeding in the gastrointestinal tract & the brain and cracking in small blood vessels.

3. Eggplant is recommended in case of gout and cardiovascular diseases.

4. Eating cherry regularly strengthens blood vessels prevents from atherosclerosis.

5. The black hawthorn juice makes it possible to recuperate for the elderly who can not even stand up, loses panting and fatigue within 10-14 days and keeps the sleep quiet. To do this, crush half a kilo of black hawthorn with a wooden spoon and add half a bowl of water. Then heat it up to 40C and make the juice pass through the cheese-cloth. Three times a day, drink a tablespoon of it before a meal.

6. Take a liter of honey and add 10 lemon water into it. Clean 10 heads of garlic, then grate and add it to your honey compound and admix them all. Preserve the prepared mixture in a sealed container for a week. Consume a teaspoon of it before a meal, three times a day so as to strengthen your heart and facilitate its muscle's work.

7. As we know that the basis of all diseases comes from nervousness, so try not to be nervous at home, at work, and in the street.

III.   Recommendations for the elderly to rejuvenate and cleanse the body:

1. Avicenna said, "If you want to keep your youthfulness, you must consume honey!" as honey contains pollen (flower dust) which positively affects the aging body. Consuming pollen itself intensifies its effects and benefits. Hence, in many countries, in a sealed container,s pollen and queen bee milk are produced excepting honey. So you must swallow dry pollen and drink water afterward. Consuming 20 grams of it daily on an empty stomach provides perfect benefits. The treatment should last for a month. Repeating it at the beginning of every season would be a great effulgence on a light.

2. Since ancient times, the carrot has been used as a means of rejuvenating and growing height. People who are highly unlikely to consume carrots age faster. Their bodies rapidly become dry, skins are wrinkled and roughened. Hair loses its color and glamor, and eyes become blurry. The teeth will soon become sore and drop one by one.

3. Low sodium diet. This diet is important for cleaning the body (especially every spring). Saltless porridge made from wheat, barley, and oats is eaten for ten days. Each spoonful should be masticated at least 25 times and

swallowed. Then nothing else is swallowed. You should drink as little water as possible.

4. Every morning you must drink the following mixture: a teaspoon of lemon juice, a teaspoon of warmed-over honey, a teaspoon of olive oil. This mixture removes toxic substances from the body, cleans the blood and brightens the face.

5. Boil a cup of milk (or water) and add 2 minced cloves of garlic to it. Take it out of the fire before boiling and then cure it for 10 minutes. The ready liquid is consumed once a week. It clears the body too.

IV.   Means for eliminating strengthlessness & weakness and strengthening the entire body:

1. Melon is the first power source. It makes the body powerful and forestalls anemia, pumps urine well, propels the viscera, and eradicates rheumatism.

2. Take a tablespoon of wheat bran and pour two bowls of water into it. Boil it for 30-40 minutes. Then add 1 tbsp of honey and boil again. Drink 50 ml 3-4 times a day. This is useful for weak children and the elderly who are ill. It strengthens the body and enhances the power.

3. Boil two tablespoons of dried rose hip in half a liter of water for 15 minutes at low heat. Cover in a thick object and cure for a night. You must drink it with honey during the day instead of tea.

4. Avicenna commands the elderly and the weak to consume fig. It also gives power to people who have lately recovered.

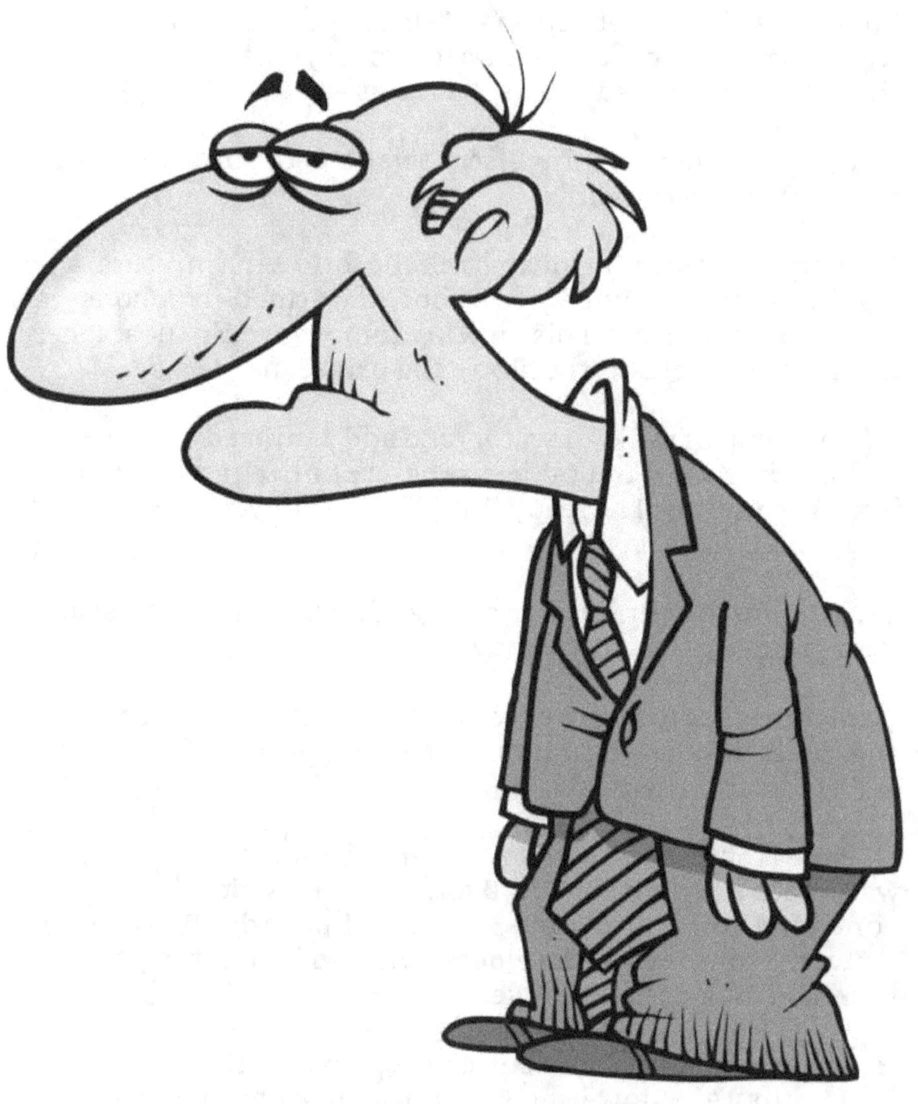

CHAPTER VII
The Viewpoint of The Wise

The following perspectives of the wise can undoubtedly help a person's longevity. As mentioned in their books, it is necessary to avoid the conversation of eight different people and to draw close to the conversation of eight different people.

The first of the eight people to escape from are those who do not know the right of salt, the second people are those who have causeless anger, the third ones are those who are proud of their longevity and consider themselves free from the rules of morality doing what pleases their heart, the fourth ones are those who execute every action with a sly scheme and find it correct, the fifth ones are those who do not admit propriety and honesty since they make lie and betrayal their motos, the sixth ones are those who yield to temptation and understand the desire as the Qibla of goal, the seventh ones are those who are shameless and spend the day with immorality and inexperience, the eighth ones are those who think bad things about good people for no reason and throw the stones of slander to contrivance of the wise without any documentation.

Conversely, the first of the eight people to approach and engage in their conversation are those who know what is kindness and do the right things, the second people are those who do not even change under all the circumstances of the period of love, the third ones are those who honor and esteem the tools that trained the great men, the fourth ones are those who are on a diet of arrogance, debauchery, and bawdiness, the fifth ones are those who can control themselves during anger, the sixth ones are those who raise the banner of favor and provide the needs of the unfortunate people, the seventh ones are those who made a shame as their own weapon so that they never go beyond the limits of morality, in any case, the eighth ones are those who foster friendships with savants & the wise and shun the immoral.

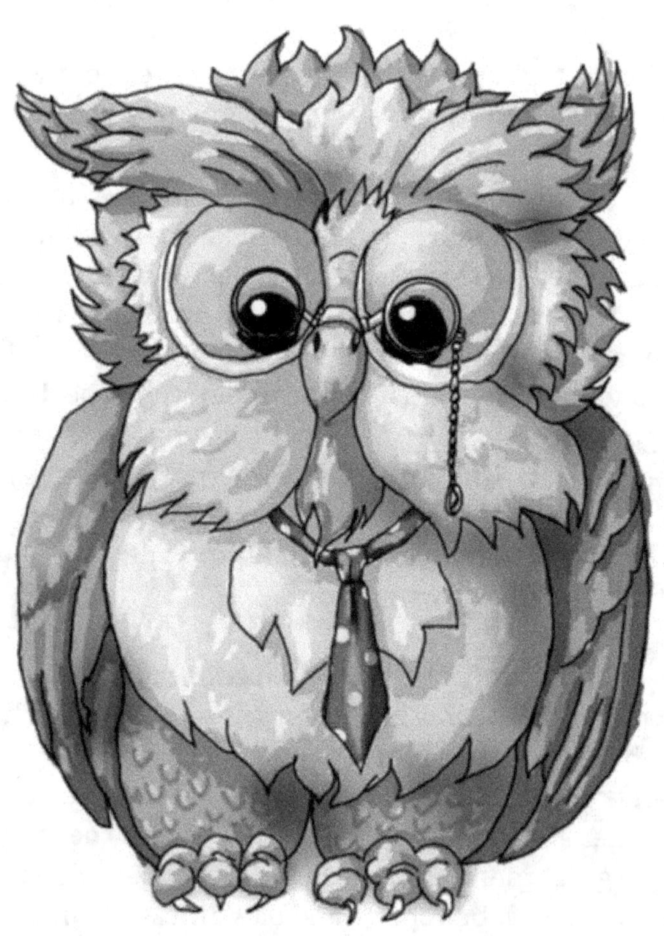

CHAPTER VIII

Appreciate Your Youthhood

The great people said wonderful words about this. In particular, the first chapter of Mevlana Husain Wais's book titled as "The Treasure of Medicine" is entitled "Nature and Man". The following words from Hafez in that book are very valuable: "O son, I read in a book: Human strength is increased every day until the age of 34. From 34 to 40 ages, human strength does not multiply or decline, it remains the same. From 40 up to 50 years of age, every year, a human begins to feel that his strength has a deficiency. Everyone at the ages of 50 to 60 goes through physical deficiency every month. Then they feel the pain everywhere on their body. The powerful peak of life is the age of 40. The slow decline starts after 40 years of age.

Oh son, here's what you understand about old age. So, always show respect to the elderly." The most beautiful and wonderful country of Japan in the world, It is also famous for its amazing people. Everything is distinctive and unique. Japanese culture is the richest in the world too. The Japanese tend to think of everything such as education, behavior, dressing, sports and even eating as an art.

Many scientists believe that the Japanese's longevity must be sought from their food menu. Japanese people have been reckoned as the longest-living people thanks to their quality food. The average life expectancy in the country is 80 years. In this respect, they are the first in the world. The main ingredient of Japanese cuisine is seafood. In addition, Japanese people are quite polite and strictly follow the rules of morality. Content is also dominant in their lives because they put discipline first. Some western scientists believe that the Japanese are long-lived because of their harmony in nicety and nature.

There is a serious attitude toward the generally accepted code of conduct in Japan: the common sense, respect for the inter-locutor, and who said that the sweet words wouldn't extend everyone's life? Of course they do! There is no doubt that the habits of punctuality, seriousness and politeness that bring luck to Japanese youth can dedicate long and meaningful life to everyone.

Scientists at the University of Ottawa (Canada) and University of Porto (Portugal) say that the limited amount of calories in food prolongs the life span. As usual, scientists experimented with mice. It turned out that the mice that were fed with low caloric food could live on average 30 percent more than they normally lived and ate. Low-calorie nutrition decelerates the organism's aging, and prevents inflammation. This is just the preliminary conclusion of the scientists.

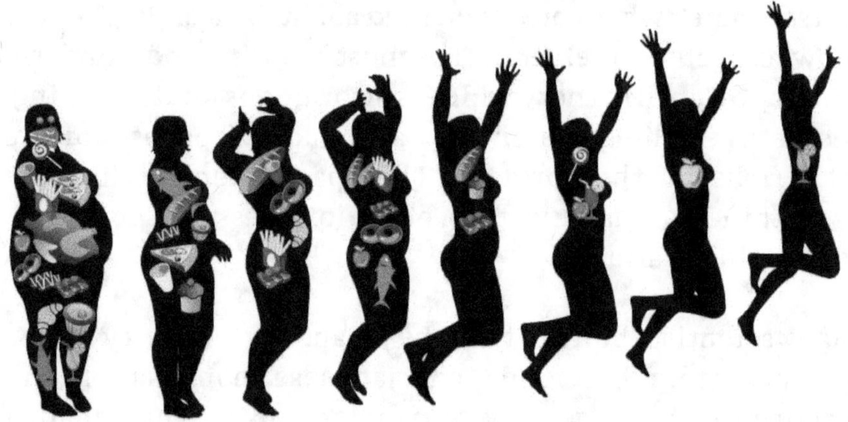

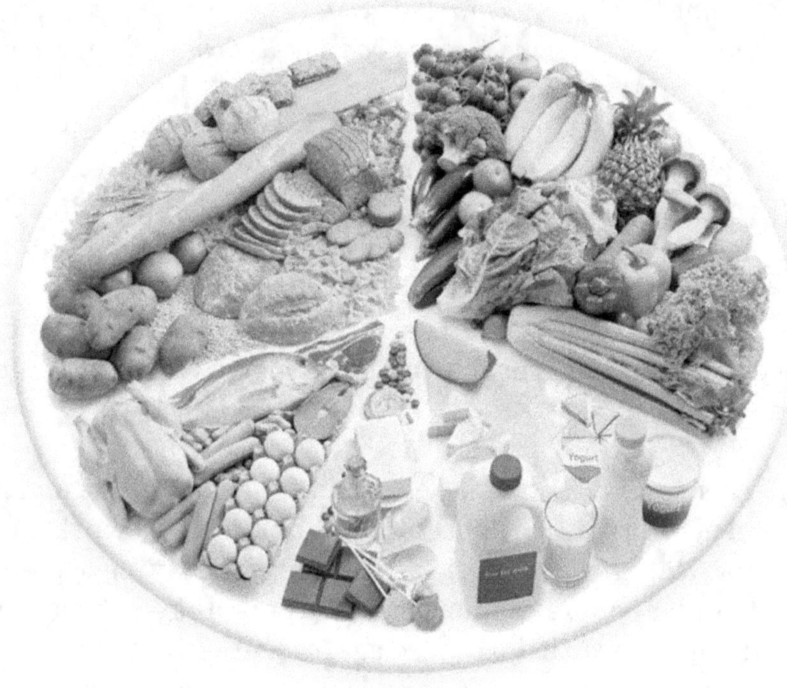

CHAPTER IX

Healthy Lifestyle-Assured Longevity

"To live a long life, a person must have proper nutrition, work hard, rest, and not be nervous and also his body needs to be hardened and sweated regularly."

(Avicenna)

Man is the highest quality of the Creator, the sublimity of nature, the corolla of life and the head of living things. Once a person comes to life, he will live and grow. He creates happiness through his work. He also makes people, his life and his society flourish. He leaves the memories if any way, they are good or bad.

The great scientist Avicenna described the health of the mature people in his work called "The Brochure about Housework" and he put physical activities in the first place while giving hygienic advice to older people. Whilst Avicenna paraphrases the maintenance of good health during old age into an active old age, he writes that the most developed and mature state is a country of long-lived people.

The science of rejuvenation and youth preservation called juvenology originated by relying on the unique ideas and scientific researches of great scientists of the past such as Hippocrates, Pavlov, Semashko, Solovieva, and others.

According to the sharpness of Avicenna's hygienic outlook and medical observation being in the prophylactic direction and his own social optimism, he can be regarded as one of the great founders of the science of juvenology which is currently being formed.

Avicenna said that by adhering "the hygienic procedures", the aging process can be managed. Modern medicine paraphrases it into "prolonging the life through a healthy lifestyle". The meaning of a healthy lifestyle includes many factors, namely the hygiene of work and vacation, proper nutrition, engagement in physical training and sports, tempering the body, adherence to sanitary culture, hygienic education of the public, etc. The chief factor of disease prevention (prophylaxis) is healthy lifestyle which is a crucial stage in the fight for the prevention of the most prevalent and severe heart disease, hypertension (myocardial infarction, stroke), oncological diseases, injuries, metabolic and mental disorders. Therefore, it is primarily dependent on ourselves to have a healthy lifestyle and to be healthy.

In the book "Medical Laws," Avicenna pointed out about the health of the elderly and called the elderly those who have moved years ahead have a great deal of expertise and wisdom. In addition to this view, modern Russian scientist I. V. Davydovsky explains: "The power" of the old man to adapt to conditions is actually diminished, but replaces it with a sense of the supremacy of knowledge, professionalism, ability, wisdom, comprehensive worldview and social responsibility. In time, a person will gain experience and become wiser, and this is a characteristic of a mature and elderly person, so young people respect and appreciate the elderly."

According to the philosopher I. V. Vishev, the huge problem of prolonging human life is not solely solved by gerontology which is the scientific study of old age, the process of aging, and the particular problems of old people. The new science Juvenology deals with the task of maintaining the life activity of an organism at a moderate level. Juvenology is closely linked to the science of gerontology and other sciences, and it develops in cooperation with them. Juvenology acknowledges the crucial and leading role of labor, especially creative work, in human life. People are able to keep the spiritual and other possibilities of youth at 60, 80, 90 or even 100 years old.

Thus, hard work is of particular importance in factors that influence the individual. Literally, the working activity of a person is his natural state, a vital condition of life. The organism can not have the required stimulus for its vital activity.

"Work creates an experience, and experience creates wisdom. They are mother and child" said Leonardo da Vinci. "Doing nothing is the misery of the elderly!" wrote 82-year- old Victor Hugo.

Leo Tolstoy answered the question of "What is happiness?" as "Happiness is   the state of a person when he fully feels his spiritual and physical strength and is able to use his working ability for the benefit of society."

All of the great people have been motivated to work and have shown love for their work. A person should be able to feel the benefits and purposefulness of his work. An inexplicable effort can only be pain and affliction. On the contrary, the hard work, but the work that aimed at improving the welfare of people purifies a person's soul and pleases him for life. A person's job dissatisfaction, nervous breakdowns, and disadvantages make life shorter. Extremely strong negative feelings may aggravate the physical and psychological weaknesses of an elderly person, causing pain in his body and causing irreparable irregularities. The old people's nerves become exquisitely sensitive, get engendered and damaged by little thing, and so, it is our duty to protect the elderly.

Cheerfulness, conviviality, amusement, and smile are essential for young people and old people to live a healthy life. Apparently, when the work starts to weary people and when they reach a certain age, they will stop their favorite work, retire, start a rest, live in peace and quiet. This factor sometimes causes a sharp change in the habit of working, causing the heart to feel lonely, and the person begins to feel isolated. Only those with a strong will can withstand such tension in life.

But we must not forget that sooner or later the retirement is inevitable. Everyone has to prepare himself beforehand for such a radical change in life.

The real man, during retirement, does not abandon his active life, and science research confirms that this is the right way. Euphoria and inspirational work are distinctive barriers to any illness, they refresh, brisk and rejuvenate a person and keep his health. Therefore, retirees should be occupied with business according to their own condition (horticulture, apiculture, mastership, tutorship, etc.).

Undoubtedly, it is difficult to get away from society and break the habit of a lifetime, and then, unfortunately, it leads to the aggravation of the aging process. It is necessary to consciously strengthen the health with plans by engaging profitable work, have the ability to be industrious and maintain thinking even in the old age. Because health is one of the most important values of society.

Keeping and strengthening it is a vital necessity and a social duty for every person in any country.

The elderly and pensioners, lonely old and disabled people and others need our support at all times. Concerning about their health and social protection is among the most important. Therefore, the material and moral support for the socially vulnerable class of the population is of particular importance in strengthening their social protection.

It is well known from the history that healthiness and longevity is the dream of humanity. From that point of view, the main task of any society is to realize this human dreams and to create conditions for the health and longevity of people. According to the World Health Organization's data and academic U. Lisitsin and B. Komarov, human health depends on the following factors, namely lifestyle - 55%, heredity (biological) - 18 %, the environment - 17%, and state of health care - 10%.

If everyone can use these factors correctly, they may be able to become guardian for their own health. Hence, the cause of many illnesses depends on a person himself. Because of the lack of sanitation in the population, unhealthy lifestyle and inadequate attention to own health, it is natural that various diseases can occur. So, our health depends largely on ourselves, or on the way we live.

According to the World Health Organization's teachings, the main trends in shaping a healthy lifestyle depend on proper nutrition, active lifestyle, and exercise, sexual education, healthy family, ensuring the spiritual well-being, avoiding harmful habits, keeping personal and public hygiene.

According to Avicenna's teachings: proper nutrition, physical fitness, proper rest, seasonal dressing, keeping safe from harmful habits, keeping the body weight normal and avoiding different tensions (stress).

According to, American scientists, Belloc and Breslow's teachings: 7-8 hours of everyday sleep, eating foods 3 times a day, daily breakfast, daily exercise, keeping the weight normal, not to consume alcohol excessively, quitting smoking. According to B. Petrenko's, a prominent medical scientist, interpretation: personal hygiene, occupational and leisure procedure, physical activity, and sweating, systematic and quality nutrition, psychohygiene and psychoprophylaxis, external environment and health, drug abuse and toxicomania, sexual education, AIDS and its prevention. Healthy lifestyle trends in the teachings of scientists and staff of the Institute of Health of the Republic of Uzbekistan:

1) Proper and rational nutrition;

2) Active life and exercise;

3) Organizing the day and working schedule on the basis of biorhythmic laws;

4) Sexual education, healthy family;

5) Ensuring the spiritual well-being;

6) Avoiding harmful habits;

7) Compliance with personal and public health;

8) Precautions for accidents and injuries;

9) Having knowledge and skills in a healthy lifestyle.

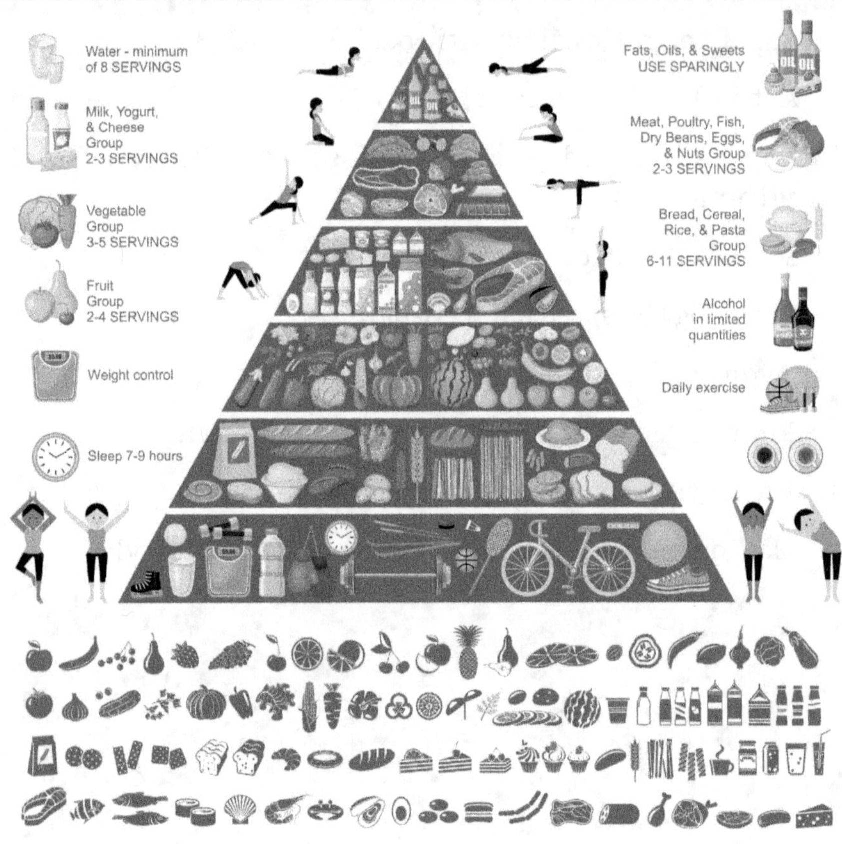

HEALTHY EATING PYRAMID
Water - minimum of 8 SERVINGS
Milk, Yogurt, & Cheese Group 2-3 SERVINGS
Vegetable Group 3-5 SERVINGS
Fruit Group 2-4 SERVINGS
Weight control
Sleep 7-9 hours
Fats, Oils, & Sweets USE SPARINGLY
Meat, Poultry, Fish, Dry Beans, Eggs, & Nuts Group 2-3 SERVINGS
Bread, Cereal, Rice, & Pasta Group 6-11 SERVINGS
Alcohol in limited quantities
Daily exercise

CHAPTER X
Springtime Illnesses

The spring season is the most beautiful and most delicate season among the seasons and is the epoch of revival and renewal of all living things on earth. Their struggle for survival, fertility, growth, and development begins mainly in the spring. That's why Avicenna said, "Spring is the best healing season of a human's life". At the same time, spring weather affects all parts of the human body such as cardiovascular, nervous, gastrointestinal, respiratory, and spinal systems, foot-to-hand, liver, kidneys, and other organs. In addition, spring has proven to cause various chronic diseases in the human body. Because the human body needs some vitamins, mineral substances, micro & macro-elements during the transition from winter to spring. The sudden change in the air (heating and cooling of the day) has a great effect on the nervous system. At this point, insomnia increases, breathing deteriorates, nervousness, high blood pressure, and headaches are observed to happen. The patients who have such troubles should drink calming drugs with the help of a physician who is supposed to reduce the blood pressure during the weather changes. The emergence of such seasonal tiredness, strengthlessness, some acute and chronic illnesses is characterized with the phrase such as "the time of ripped marrow" or "human energy goes to trees".

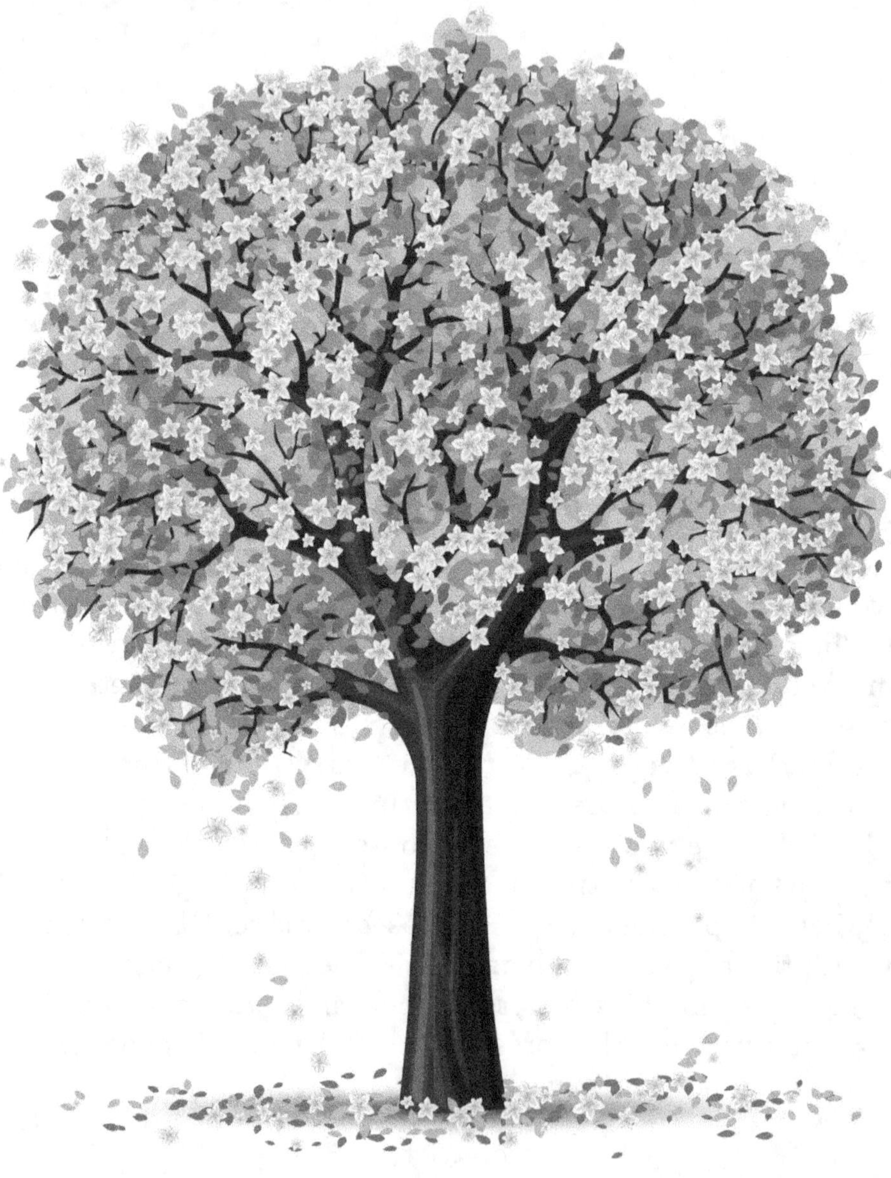

That's why every person and family should be able to do a number of activities starting from the spring in order to be healthy throughout the year:

1. Shepherd's purse, sorrel, mint, plantain, dandelion, trefoil, nettle, spinach, and others should be eaten in early spring.

2.   Consuming different national dishes such as dumpling, bread, samsa and liquid dishes made from medicinal herbs such as parsley, dill, basil, leek, garlic, and others is beneficial to blood.

3.   In the early spring, consuming certain types of herbs (from 15 to 30 days) increases the curativeness of the food (strength, quality, taste, the richness of beneficial substances), cleanses the blood and the internal organs of the human body and provides essential nutrients.

4.   It is recommended to grow different types of grain (wheat, barley, etc.), cook them to prepare different salads and eat them.

5.   It is recommended to eat dumpling made from 9 or 11 flowers of peach and the first minced leaves of the vine so as to avoid illness until the next spring, purify the blood and clear the faces.

6.   A person who is wearing a superficial garment may get cold in a frequently changing spring weather. Therefore, the wearing of such clothing should be light, warm and seasonal. Especially, keeping the head, body, and feet from cool and wind is significantly important.

7.   In order for the body to respond and quickly adapt to the weather changes, the person should be well-sweated from the childhood (air, water, solar baths, exercise, sports, etc.).

8.   Do not forget that the child who has been sweated, cured and well-groomed with a doctor's advice will be resistant to illness, such as colds and others.

9.   Keep in mind that the milk of the cows, sheeps, goats, horses, and camels which was fed with herbage in the spring is rich in vitamins and that the person who drinks it can quickly adapt to the spring conditions.

10.   Those who are indifferent to winter-summer herbs, fruits and vegetables, milk and dairy products become sick that they even sleep on beds and do not wake up. Then doctors are required to send medicines, vitamins, and glucose to the body of these patients.

When the spring breeze touches the chest, a person feels exhilarated, his soul rejoices and he saturates the breath. The wise say, "It's better to be in pure air than to eat medicine.

"During this time, oxidation processes in the body naturally develop. Cells can grow freely and a man enjoys the human breath and natural awakening. The blue sky and green grass make the nerves more relaxed.

CHAPTER XI
Summer and Health

"Summer melts and dissipates too much, weakens the strength and natural effects. The blood, phlegm, bile, and psoriasis increase in the summer."

(Avicenna)

Summer is the season of ripening that satisfies the needs of the body's nutrients by consuming fruits and vegetables. This season has its own concerns.

In this season, the person's body temperature rises and he begins to feel some kind of misery. It is known that the human body temperature is about 36.5 degrees. It discharges heat mainly through the skin and the lungs(breath). Scientists believe that if the heat is not discharged through the skin and lungs, the body will reach its boiling level in 40 hours. Therefore, if the air temperature is high, the body begins to heat up, a person feels uncomfortable and has trouble in breathing, thirst is felt and there will be a decrease in the amount of water and mineral salts in the human body during hot days. Air pressure drops and oxygen deficiency occurs in the human body. The great scientist, the sultan of the science of medicine, Avicenna, proved that during the hot days of the summer, the human body often develops anemia, fever, erysipelas, and other ailments due to malnutrition and poor functioning of the gastrointestinal system.

According to Avicenna's writings, the conditions like a decrease in blood pressure, headache, dizziness, dyspnea, weakness, asthenia, decreased memory, anxiety, acceleration of heartbeat and colds on legs are dependent on cardiovascular diseases. Vomiting is evident especially when a person is thirsty. As a result, the person's ability to work quickly falls and the body's heat gets worse. As a result of the observations and experiments conducted by scientists regarding the effect of summer heat on the body, it was determined that hot temperature changes the normal functioning of the body's total physiological systems.

In the cerebral cortex cells, the braking process is intensified. This may be the reason why the person who engages in a single job snoozes. Scholars claim that the function of many internal secretory glands is also changed by the effect of external temperatures. In particular, the function of the pituitary and adrenal glands increases, and the function of thyroid and sex gland decreases. It is well known that during hot days, the appetite of the person is not good, consumed food passes through the intestines slowly and stays there for a long time. Consequently, during hyperthermia (the condition of having a body temperature greatly above normal), the activity of the digestive organs, as well as the water-salt and other metabolisms in the body, are destructed and the occurrence of acute gastrointestinal disorders is observed.

Scientists have examined the tempo of physiological processes in the seasons and found that the thermal resistance of the person increases in summer and decreases in winter. The consumption of food during the thermal adaptation is significantly reduced, and the glucose and cholesterol levels drop in the blood. The human body is complicated, it needs proteins, fats, carbohydrates, and vitamins to function normally. Only if these substances are in precise balance, a person feels exhilarated. It is recommended to use meat, fish, liver, eggs, milk and dairy products, fruits, gourds and vegetables, and legumes for the body to receive the full and high-quality substances.

Many people swim in the summertime in different pools relaxing and blackening in the sunshine. It's good. As Avicenna pointed it out that the benefit of the sunlight for the body is great. The weak effect of it stimulates cells and enhances their function. Only when its light is used in the rhythm, red blood cells and hemoglobin increase in blood. It satisfies the organism's oxygen demand, improves the function of the nervous system and the muscles.

Too much sun exposure is noxious to a person. The sharp light of the sun can cause skin cells to die, damage, or develop cancer. The skin will turn red due to an increase in blood flow. It is particularly important for people who have cardiovascular, thyroid, liver, kidney and other disorders and infirm, weak and obese people, infants and the elderly to avoid the harmful effects of a sunbeam. In the broiling weather, a person can have headaches & dizziness, get lethargic, may vomit, his mouth dries, thirst increases and cheeks redden. Pulsing and breathing accelerate, unpleasant pain occurs around the heart. At a light condition of broiling weather, the body temperature is 37.5 degrees and but at a heavy one, it goes up to 39-41 degrees.

If a person sits in a muggy room or his roommate is a chain-smoker, even if he wears synthetic clothes in hot days, the heat can expose him. Here, too, is the condition as heatstroke, the pulse increases, the feet and hands tremble, the face reddens and the heartbeat and breathing accelerate, and the body temperature rises to 38-40 degrees. In severe heatstroke, a person may lose consciousness, cease breathing, the heartbeat may stop as well. When giving the first aid to the person who experienced heatstroke, it is necessary to quickly take him to shade. At such a moment, it is important to call an ambulance or take the patient to the hospital immediately.

Until the ambulance comes, a patient's face is washed with cold water, his body is wiped with a wet towel, and ice or moistened cloth is put on his forehead. If the patient is conscious, he should drink cold water (half a teaspoon of salt in a glass of water). Sometimes small cotton is adsorbed in sal-ammoniac and smelled so that it is easy to breathe. If the patient is unconscious and the pulse is not felt, artificial respiration given. It is also necessary to massage the heart of a sick person.

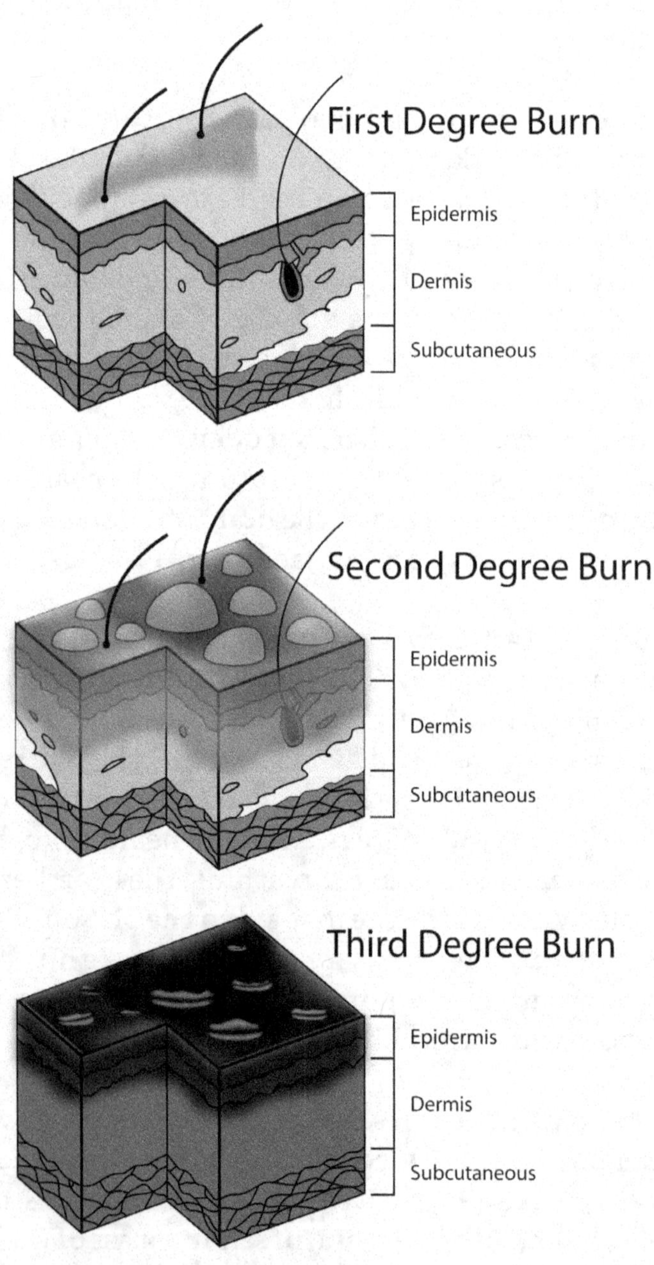

To avoid such unpleasantness, some of the following recommendations are referred to you:

1. Wear preferable outer garment which is naturally fibrous, broader, light, fine, and white. Fashionable fabrics do not make the air pass.

2. Fat food and sweets should not be consumed too much. It is beneficial to eat more vitamins such as fruits, vegetables, greens, sour cream soups (eg, mastava, moshxo'rda, qaynatma sho'rva, ugra osh, etc.:)).

3. Do not drink plenty of water when you are thirsty, instead, drink green tea, different fruit and vegetable juices, compote, kvass, and buttermilk.

4. It is unhealthy to immediately drink cold water, tea, and juice or eating ice cream after consuming hot food and tea.

5. After blackening under the sun, it is necessary to have some rest in the shade, then bathe or shower, be wiped with a wet towel. Jumping over into cold water results in cold and vascular stretch when sweating.

If everyone puts work and rest in the right way, consumes quality foods, follows to sanitary-cum-hygienic rules (cleanliness) and aforesaid recommendations, they will spend the summer and its hot days without any troubles.

CHAPTER XII

The Risk of Autumn Cold

The weather of autumn often changes. It's cool in the evenings and breezy in the mornings, it rains as well. In such weather conditions, a person can get cold, suffer sniffle or influenza. At the same time, selfishly using various medicines can lead to dangerous illnesses.

Avicenna described the nature of the autumn as: "In autumn, people walk under the hot sun, walk out at the cold in the evening, there are a lot of illnesses due to the plentiness of fruits, spoiling of mucus and loss of energy during the summer.

Although the months of early autumn are somewhat favorable for older people, the end results as unfavorable.

The autumn diseases are as follows: tetter, herpes, cancerous tumors, joint pains, fever, and so on. The reason for all this is the abundance of yellow bile. In the autumn, lung diseases, hip and back pains are increased, this is because poops move in the summer and compress in autumn. The best autumn is the rainy and wet one, the dry one is the worst one".

According to researchers, colds are mostly caused by inflammation of the upper respiratory tract such as rhinitis (inflammation of the mucous membrane of the nose, caused by a virus infection (e.g., the common cold) or by an allergic reaction (e.g., hay fever)), pharyngitis (inflammation of the pharynx, causing a sore throat), laryngitis (inflammation of the larynx, typically resulting in huskiness or loss of the voice, harsh breathing, and a painful cough), tracheitis (inflammation of the trachea, usually secondary to a nose or throat infection) and bronchitis (inflammation of the mucous membrane in the bronchial tubes. It typically causes bronchospasm and coughing). The most sensitive organs to the cold and heats are legs and upper respiratory tract. If the legs get cold, the temperature in the body decreases and this affects the upper respiratory tract, which results in the cold. Therefore, in the cool and cold weather of the year, the legs should be kept warm first. The flu is usually accompanied by a sneeze, throat pain, nasal flow, exhaustion, loss of mood, headache or dizziness. Occasionally, fl including influenza can be observed by pain in eyelashes, vertigo and high temperature in the body. If the above-mentioned symptoms appear, it is important to seek medical advice immediately.

Here are some of the simplest and harmless treatments recommended by folk and modern medicines and used by the majority of people as home treatments when severe coughing occurs:

1. when you get cold, consume a spoonful of butter putting it in boiling milk or milk with baking soda (about in a bowl of milk, in ratio, half a teaspoonful of baking soda) in order to soften the throat, leave cough behind and get rid of phlegm easily. And also cooking quince and turnip putting butter or buttock between them helps a dry cough.

2. Infuse 20 grams of chopped jujube fruits with a half teapot of boiling water for an hour. Drink the infusion three times a day, 50 grams before eating. The infusion gives a positive effect to upper respiratory tracts, but also relieves a dry cough and facilitates phlegm removal.

3. The infusion of fig and dandelion softens the throat, lowers fever, discharges sweat and removes phlegm.

4. During the onset of the flu, frequent smelling of chopped onion or garlic prevents the onion or garlic prevents the pain from deterioration.

5. Onion juice is useful during cough and bronchitis. For this, boil 500 grams of chopped onion, 50 grams of honey, 40 grams of sugar and 1 liter of water for 3 hours on light flame. Then the

mixture is cooled and put in a well-covered container. Drink a tablespoon out of the juice 4-5 times a day. Equal amounts of onion, apple, and honey are mixed.

6. Consuming 2-3 teaspoons 2-3 times a day can prevent from throat inflammation.

7. Drink hot water during a headache. Eat just two cloves of garlic. Put cabbage leaves on your forehead.

8. When the patient's temperature is high, drinking tea with lemon and during coughing, breathing difficulties and chest pains, drinking tea with blackberry and raspberry help the patient improve his condition, reduce headaches and lower fever.

9. Peganum is disinfectant and it can be advantageous if kept in a patient's room.

10. It is efficient for a patient to eat foods filled with greens, vegetables, and various vitamins as much as possible.

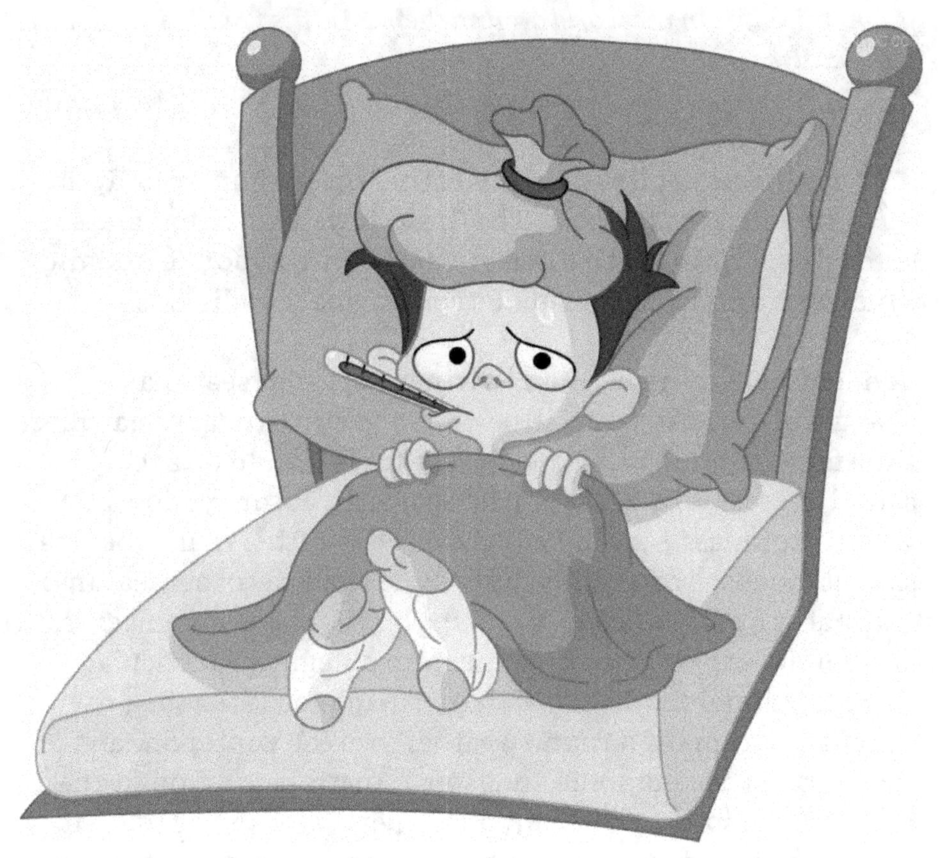

CHAPTER XIII
Serious Diseases of Winter

"Seasons of the year can vary significantly in characteristics and prompt changes in the world around them... If this breaks, it will cause serious diseases."

(Avicenna)

The effects of climate and weather on the human body are known from the past. The Greek physician Hippocrates started describing each illness in his writings about epidemic illnesses from the effects of meteorological conditions.

Avicenna writes in his own writings that "The seasonal changes of year cause any illness in each climate. The healthiest time for autumn is rainy and for winter it should be as cold as a mild degree. Winter is the best season to absorb yellow bile with its coldness, long night and short day rather than other seasons. It hides the bad yellow biles more than any other seasons and makes a person needy for taking lenitives and demulcents. Most of the winter diseases come from phlegm. In particular, there are numerous diseases alike with influenza that begin with the change from the autumn weather into the winter one and then turn into pneumonia, lung inflammation, and frog-in-the-throat. Then spinal pains can appear, nerves become damaged, a prolonged headache can be triggered, and even stroke and epilepsy may appear.

That all emanates from fatigue and the proliferation of phlegm". During the frosty days of winter, various types of colds such as fever, bronchitis, angina, pleurisy, influenza, pneumonia increase. Ways to fight colds are simple: a person must prepare the body for the sharp changes in weather, for example, the body should be sweated and, most importantly, it should be kept from the cold not wearing superficial clothes. In the winter months, the atmospheric temperature is about 8-10 degrees from heat and 5-10 degrees to cold. The aging power of the organism is not so adapted to such a temperature since skin veins are narrowed. As a result, circulation in the blood vessels destructs, a decrease in heat is observed at the layer of skin. Scientists emphasize that lowering the temperature in the skin tissues reduces the supply of oxygen by arterial blood vessels. As a result, the muscle of some organs and nerve fibers get cold. It is known that fever is associated with colds and inflammation of the upper respiratory tract. In the first case, a patient can have painful headaches, sneeze, throat pain, rhinorrhea, giddiness, pains around eyelids and eyebrows are observed. If an acute fever repeats often, it can turn to chronic. It is known that this is mostly caused by smoking, alcohol abuse, constipation, heart and kidney diseases. It is absolutely wrong for the patient to be cured as he knows that fever is a mild disease.

Influenza is the most infectious and dangerous diseases of winter, and it has a rapidly spreading effect. In 1933, British scientists discovered that viruses play a major role in the origination of influenza. Multiple viral particles falling into the cells of respiratory passages are found to multiply to more than one billion under favorable conditions during one day.

As a result, the patient can spread influenza viruses to healthy people by coughing, sneezing and speaking. After viruses have multiplied, they excrete toxic substances, intoxicate the body, disrupt the brain function and nervous system, make the symptoms of lethargy, cluster headaches, sweating, coughing, sciatica, weakness, insomnia, sore throat, and anorexia appear. Most of the time a patient gets flu, in most cases, a dry cough and sneeze are seen to arise. If the patient does not receive treatment timely, the effect of influenza can produce a number of complications in the lungs and organs. Influenza can also result in pneumonia which inflames the bronchi and nasal cavity. The inflammation of the brain and cortex extremely dangerous complications of influenza. The patient should be treated only under the supervision of a physician, only then the complications can be prevented.

Pneumonia disturbs during the winter months and low temperatures, especially, weak people who do not perspire their body. The pneumonic disease occurs in people of all ages. Its origin is primarily due to factors such as having the body which has not been hardened to external temperatures, not wearing seasonally, excessive fatigue, not following the procedures of eating, working and resting.

Depending on the passage of the disease, it is differed as acute and chronic; depending on the place, it is differed as in the limited types and bronchopneumonia or lobular pneumonia. Acute pneumonia begins suddenly, fever rises, when breathing and coughing, thorax hurts. During lobular pneumonia, a patient coughs and spits phlegm, and his temperature goes up to 38-40 degrees. Chronic pneumonia has proven to be a cause of damage to the bronchi, pulmonary veins, and lymphatic system. If pneumonia is not treated timely, it often results in any complications, such as the accumulation of water in the lungs, the chronic inflammation of the lung, tuberculosis and the narrowing of the respiratory ducts.

Angina is contagious and associated with colds as well. If the disease is not timely treated, it binds heart with pain and causes other organs to be hurt. People of all ages should be provided with powerful foods that are pleasing to them during the appearance of diseases associated with colds namely influenza, angina, pneumonia and others. Because the body parts of the patient are in dire need of vitamins.

Drinking infusion made from rosehips is essential not only for the patients but also for healthy people that increases the body's resistance to infectious diseases and intensifies its protection. Medications should be used only when prescribed by the doctor for various types of colds. Normally giving more liquids, fruit and vegetable juices (such as apple, fig, cherry, pomegranate, orange, blackberry, raspberry, carrot, beet, etc.) to the patient who has been infected with influenza is beneficial to the blood.

It is recommended for a patient to consume lightly formative foods for his body parts. Peppers and kinds of vinegar should not be added to patients' meals and they should not smoke or drink alcohol. In order not to catch colds, everyone needs to sweat and strengthen themselves, especially, keep the feet and head warm.

The separate room where the patient sleeps should be bright, full of air, not be above 25 degrees and peganum harmala should be burnt frequently, the perfume should be sprayed as well. During the influenza attack, raspberry jam tea can be used to sweat the body, relieve pain, lower the temperature and everyday, before eating, mixing sliced onions with sour cream (add 1 tbsp of sour cream to 1 tbsp of onion) along with eating 2-3 pieces of garlic 2-3 times a day are beneficial for the blood. It also has many positive effects if a decoction of figs is consumed and also a spoonful of honey mixed with butter is swilled with a teaspoon.

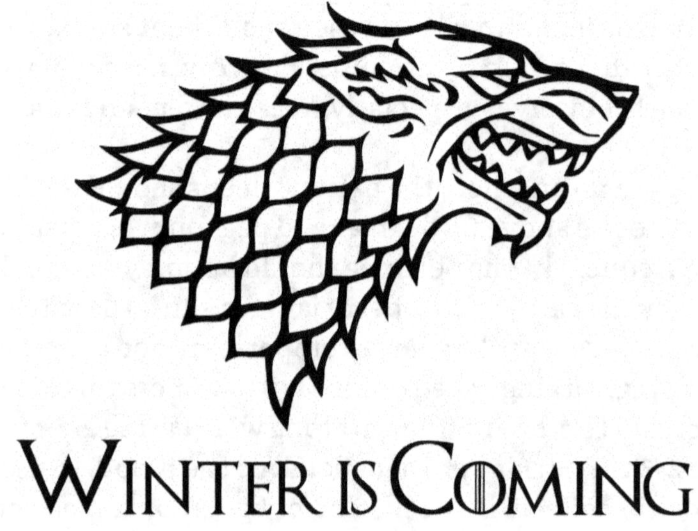
WINTER IS COMING

CHAPTER XIV
Dignity-Adornment of Life

"The precious moments of our precious age
Ask dear people for dignity.
An opportunity is transient,
It is time to decorate the book of life."
(Gafur Gulom)

A man strives for perfection throughout his life. He creates his own life and happiness according to his ability and contributes to the development of society. As a result, he brings up children who will continue his work. He finds dignity due to his virtues. Keeping healthiness throughout the life decorates the meaning of life.

Showing worth is highly glorified by our people. Valuing the parents is both duty and debt. Appreciating the elderly is a great attribute. Showing worth to invalids, lonely people, orphans, widows and the poor is the greatest blessing. There are many types of dignity to be shown to the family, by the husband to wife, by the wife to husband, neighbors, and neighborhood. Its value and meanings are measured by the dignity of the person. Indeed, as long as a person lives, only his virtues will remain. Generations do not estimate according to how many years he lived, but according to his good deeds.

Honor and attention to the elderly and posterity is a perpetual custom in our nation. Nowadays, the contribution of our elderly people to the material, spiritual and cultural development of the country is widely supported and promoted. Their life experiences are an invaluable treasure and exemplary school for our young people. In the cities & villages, schools & lyceums, colleges & universities, thereupon, meetings are being held with grandparents who are well-known for their sapiential works. These events, in turn, raise the spirit of our elderly people and they are once again feeling that they are useful and needful to our society.

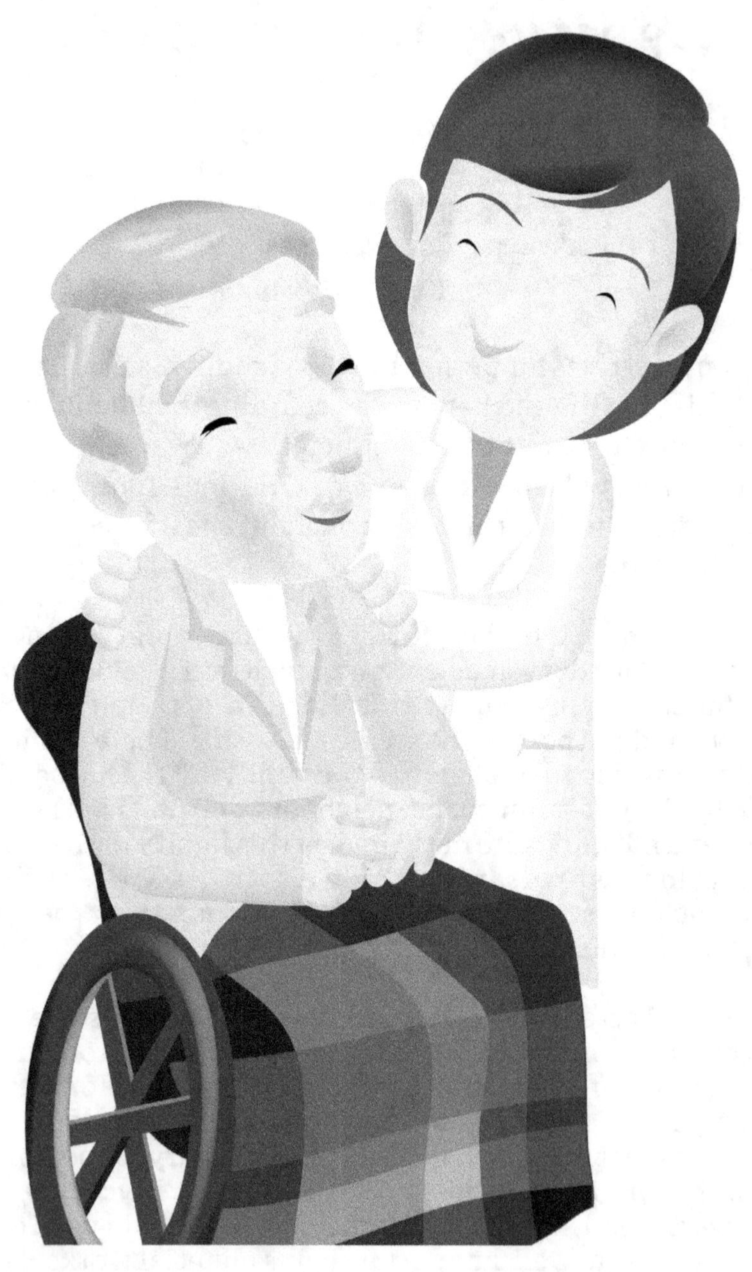

CHAPTER XV

Honey Prolongs Youthfulness

Since ancient times, honey, propolis (bee glue), royal jelly (bee milk) and apitoxin (bee venom) have been widely used as a treatment for various diseases in folk medicine as it contains more than 100 biologically active substances needed by the human body, the most important of which are carbohydrates, enzymes, vitamins, and minerals.

According to Avicenna's book called "Laws of Medicine", honey affords refreshment, improves digestion, removes phlegm, heals inflammation, strengthens remembrance and prolongs youthfulness. According to Avicenna, particularly those who are over 45 years of age need to consume honey with nuts.

For example, honey gives power during weakness, fatigue, and tuberculosis. To do this, it is recommended to drink a fresh carrot juice or milk with honey about 60 and 100 grams per day. It provides good results if the people who experience sleep deprivation at night consume a spoonful of honey every day before dinner. It is also used as a power-enhancing agent for sexual inefficiency. In this case, an onion is ground on the pestle and its water is squeezed. Then it is cooked until it has slowly flowed onto a low heat, adding honey to it. The prepared product is consumed two to three spoonfuls every night.

Some people suffer leg cramp in the night and awake due to pain. It can also be treated with honey. Each time you eat two teaspoons of honey before eating, that's it, you will be cured in a week.

Using natural honey of mountain with carrot juice during a bronchial cough associated with the upper respiratory tract inflammation gives a positive result. If given 1 tbsp of honey, before going to bed, to the children who are so used to moistening in the bed while sleeping, the result can be effective.

Royal jelly can be used to treat bronchial asthma, bronchitis, tracheitis, parotitis, acute and chronic inflammation, influenza, anemia, blood pressure, blood, heart,

nerves, atherosclerosis, gastrointestinal tract, liver, skin, headache, migraine, ocular diseases, and others.

Royal jelly is useful for scalp and hair care and is also used in facial skin treatments.

However, royal jelly is not recommended for use in the treatment of acute infectious and kidney disease. Among the patients there can be seen the people who have hypersensitivity to royal jelly. Some people may experience sleep deprivation, coughing or poisoning after consuming royal jelly. In such cases, it is canceled immediately.

Apitoxin has a strong antibiotic property and various creams, and ointments are prepared with the aqueous & oil-based solutions of bee honey. Bee venom and its lotions are used to treat rheumatism, tropical ulcer, the cold in brain and nerves, inflamed gums, abscess, high blood pressure, nervous system, cardiovascular and ocular diseases, and others. Patients are "stung" by a honey bee so as to treat hypertension, headaches, and asthma. According to scientists, the treatment is held in two stages. The first stage of treatment is ten days and during this period a patient is stung by 55 bees. The second stage is that a patient must be stung by 150 bees for one and a half months. The patient should be examined first whether he has an allergy to bee venom or not. Bee venom cannot be consumed by the people who have pancreas, tuberculosis, diabetes, fatigue, heart, liver, kidney and infectious diseases and various tumors.

Smoking or alcohol use is prohibited during treatment. It is unrecommended to use bee venom after eating, after water treatments or after a walk. Herbal and dairy products should be used at the time of treatment.

The propolis is used for the treatment of skin diseases, simple and chronic wounds, gastrointestinal wounds, hemorrhoids, colds, neuritis, radiculitis, and some gynecological issues. It has a positive effect on healthy people, it refreshes them and relieves lassitude.

Hippocrates advised putting a wax layer on the head and neck during the throat pains. Pliny writes that beeswax has the ability to soften intestines, heat up and restore the body. Cosmetic products (such as creams, lipsticks, etc.) are often made from beeswax. Beeswax sweet for human beings is very beneficial, it increases the function of the blood, muscle, and metabolism. Further, wax cleans teeth and strengthens gums and also helps to quit smoking.

Pollen is recommended during physical tension, anemia, memory loss, headache, insomnia, and the patient's healing. Pollen often stores the properties of plants. Knowing the pollen content, it can be possible to extract a variety of medicinal composites necessary for health. Pollen should not be consumed more than normally. Otherwise, it leads to metabolic destruction in the body. Therefore, it is unnecessary to eat honey products for a definite period of time after healing with pollens. According to medical experts, it is unrecommended to use pollens for healthy children.

According to scientists, only one apitherapy medical center

has been established in the world, for now, that is in Romania. The apitherapy center treats patients with honey bee products, including honey, pollen, beeswax, propolis, royal jelly, and bee venom.

As a result of an in-depth study, medical people have developed more effective treatment methods, namely, Apiphytotherapy (phyto- of a plant) is a new branch of medicine, herein, honey bee and plant products are used in combination. Nowadays there are more than 20 medicines made from honey bee and plant products in the country.

According to the information, chronic hepatitis, anemia, rheumatism, hypertension and many other diseases are being treated successfully by using this method.

Now in many Romanian cities, first of all, apitherapy departments have been opened at the university centers and patients are being helped.

In summary, people should not think that the honey bee products are a cure to a thousand one pains as the use or consumption of some may lead to some complications.

Therefore, a physician who recommends these products is required in the thorough examination of a patient and supervision during treatment. Patients cannot be treated without the advice of a physician and his clear guidelines.

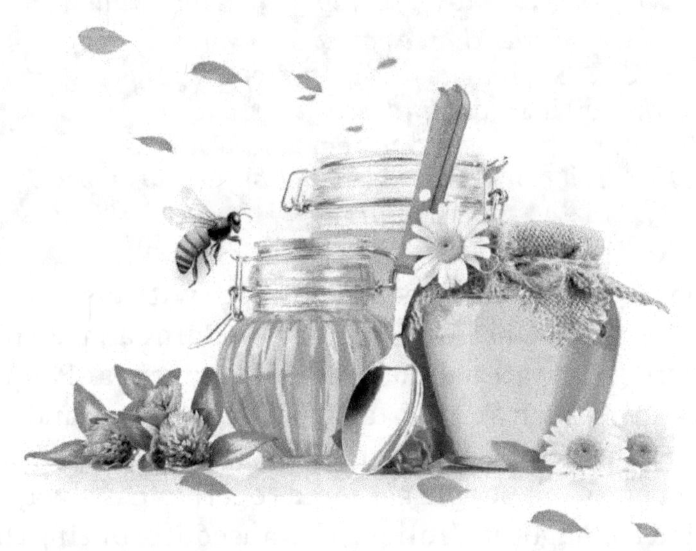

CHAPTER XVI

Extending Life with Laughter

"Giving the laugh to an unhappy one, Know that,
is better than a pound of sugar.
Mouth & tongue find taste from sugar,
But the spirit & soul find pleasure from laughter.
Your face looks sad and dark as the night,
Laugh like the morn, let wrinkles and conflicts disappear."
(Jami)

Our people have always been dabblers to witticism. Especially in the national holiday, wedding and hospitality, humorists exhilarate the audience with touches of humor and wisecracks. In such a circle, lassitude is forgotten and fair laughter gives people spiritual power as a medicine. That is why the place where people gathered together has always accompanied by laughter, drollery, and anecdote. During the Stagnation Period, some officials who were diagnosed with the diseases of management and careerism had reckoned a laugh in front of the prestigious people as a sign of remnant and incivility in public and even in recreational places.

Thanks to Independence, in the line of our national values, there have been rebuilt our witticism and humorous songs. The laughter regave attraction to our tea-houses and amusement parks.

But there is also a norm in laughter and witticism, therefore, to know how, when, where and around whom to laugh is a sign of high spirituality and culture.

It is well known from the earliest years that laughter serves as an incentive power for life, health, beauty, and emotion, as power for unleashing from pain, sorrow and sadness. Our wise people characterized it as "the laughter is the deficient healing of health, the flower of the mien". Laughing with the whole body is a natural necessity for a human body as water and air. The great scientists emphasized that If there is no joy and fun, the nous may blunt and then weaken.

Indeed, when a person laughs his heart out, it improves his health, relieves the body, refreshes the spirit, increases appetite and extends life. Famous witticist Yusufkhan Shakarjonov said that "Laugh, friends, your life will be long!". Laughter affects the whole body and increases the physical activity level. A person's mood rises from laugh. According to the scientific research of physiologists, as a result of laugh and joy, size of gastric mucus dwindles, the action of undulate enlargement and narrowing intensifies and the food is quickly digested.

Also, laughter primarily gives a zest to the brain since when a person laughs, the facial muscles contracts and the venous blood flow in the head runs smoothly. Oxygenated and nutrient-rich blood flow in arterial vessels does not change.

As a result, the pressure in the capillaries increases, and the brain is better supplied with blood. More importantly, laughter accelerates the movement of the impulse in the cerebral cortex. This helps to receive new information and reclaim it timely. As a result, the brain does not tire and tense. Additionally, laughter helps the lungs improve air exchange, increase the person's ability to work and strengthen the will. Moreover, the respiratory organs are activated since laughter starts with deep inhaling and the breath is exhaled during "hah, ha, ha".

Many scientists believe that the expansion of the thorax, just like a pump, pulls the blood of the head and decreases the blood pressure in the veins. Laughter activates these changes and improves blood flow, in other words, it massages the brain and internal organs. That's the reason why a person can relax and refresh the spirit after laughing. One of the key components that makes a person laugh with pleasure and gives him spiritual nourishment is satire. Here are some helpful tips that you can use: Habituate to the accessible and inoffensive jocosity. Read more about satires, anecdotes, and funny stories. Just relax satisfiedly by means of frequently listening to the interesting radio broadcasting and telefilms which gives you a good mood. Have fun, get rid of moody events and have at least half an hour every day to get spiritual rest and forget about the diseases altogether. Always remember Avicenna's words that "At the moment when a patient laughs, he will be a hundred percent healthy person!".

Mood changes vary from person to person but try some of these activities to find out what makes you most happy.

Science Says You Have Time For
HAPPINESS

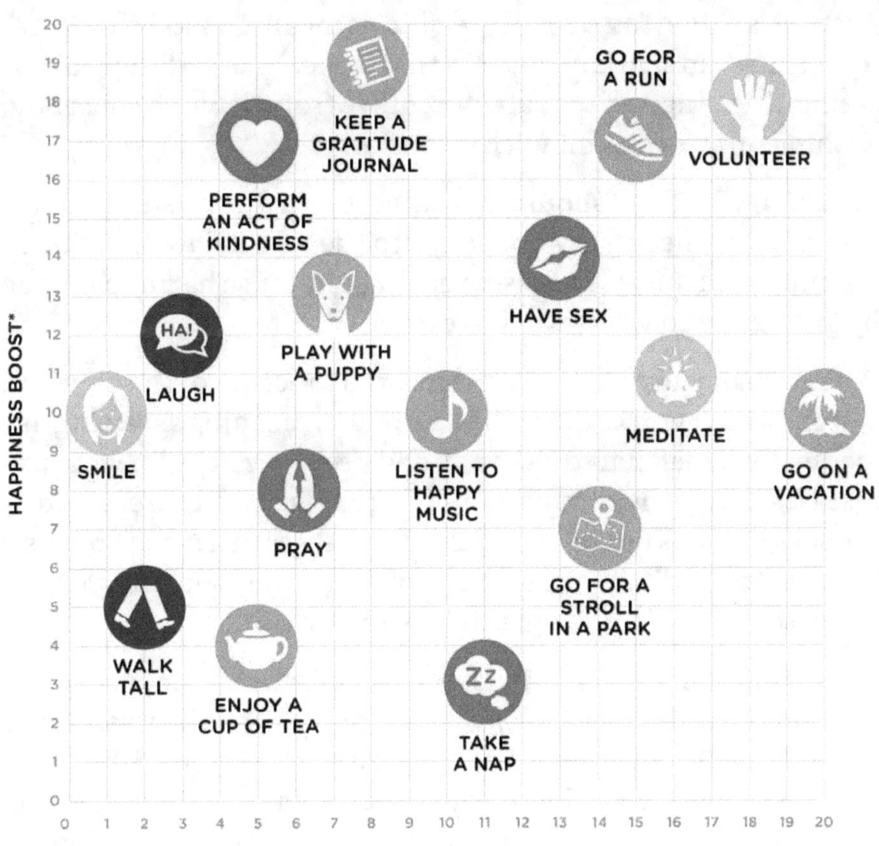

CHAPTER XVII
Fasting and Health

Fasting has been existent as spiritual education and physical worship since ancient times.

The holy month of Ramadan is sacred to all Muslims in our daily lives.

Fasting is called "as-savm" in Arabic. It means "Abstaining from something". In shariah, it is said that it means "Abstaining from eating, drinking and sexual intercourse from dawn to sunset by wishing Allah's consent with intention".

A person who fasts should also adhere to its duty, sunna and decency. It is necessary not to eat to the full at dawn, not to eat too much at sunset. Excessive eating can cause harm to human by giving rise to various diseases.

The annual pause in the uninterrupted function of the digestive system which works more than 12 hours, meaning as fasting, is medically beneficial to the body and keeps it safe from various diseases that is the fact, herein, the proof is not required. Modern science does not deny it too. Scientists say that the body is adapted to a radically changed provision order within a month, increases the ability to fight illness and so on.

The French doctor recommends that everyone over the age of 40 should stay hungry every week. Prof. Y. S. Nikolaev researches more than 30 widespread diseases nowadays. The well-known Egyptian physician, a doctor of medicine, Muhammad Jafar, recommended not to fast for the patients with one of the following diseases:

1. Tuberculosis, anemia, whooping-cough, lung and heart diseases;
2. Gastrointestinal diseases;

3.   Fever, hypertension, and hypotension;
4.   For patients who have recently recovered, been in operation and are physically weak;
5.   Mothers who breastfeed, the pregnant and the elderly.

In addition to the above, it is recommended not to fast for some people with the following illnesses or some of the healthy people:
1. Patients with small intestine and colon diseases;
2.   Patients with metabolic disorders, in particular, diabetes mellitus;
3.   People who have been exhausted for a long time due to chronic illness;
4.   Young children and people who are busy with heavy physical work throughout the day.

It is better for the fasting person to consume foods which are light, nutritious and helpful for boosting power, including nut roll, whole wheat, millet, and unleavened bread, honey, dried apricot, butter or yogurt, milky foods, and steamed meals...

Iftar dishes should not be too heavy for a person who has been a hungry whole day. These comprise low fats, milky foods, home-made plov, cream of rice and soups, wet and dried fruits, vege-tables and greens.

It is noxious to the blood for a person to guzzle food at dawn and especially at sunset if he has been hungry all day.

Therefore, at dawn and sunset, 20 minutes before eating (before starting and after breaking a fast), it is best to consume a bowl of water or various wet fruits and vegetables, the digestive, to wit, foods rich in vitamins, minerals and micronutrients frequently".

If a person fasts by following above-mentioned rules, he will cer-tainly be able to recover from some illnesses.

Holy Month of Ramadan

No Eating Or Drinking Whilst Fasting

Lower Your Gaze

No Arguing Or Fighting & Avoid Sins

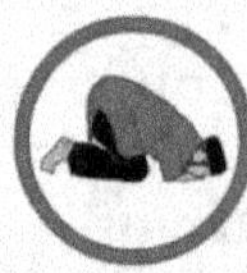

Pray All Your 5 Daily Salaah's On Time

Study & Learn Islamic Knowledge

Recite & Learn The Holy Qur'aan

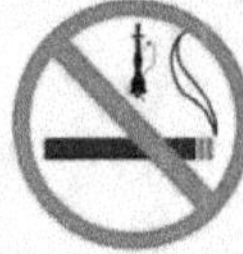

No Smoking Try Quitting For Good

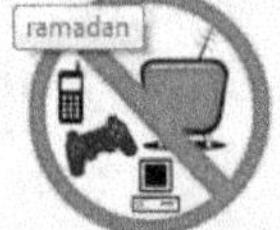

Don't Waste Time On Useless Activities

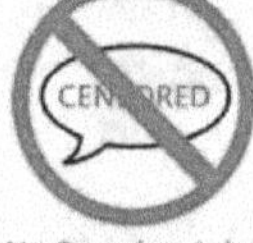

No Swearing, Lying & Backbiting

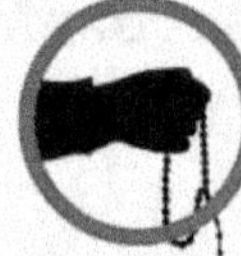

Do Lots Of Dhikr

Make Lots Of Duaa

Give In Charity & Help The Poor

CHAPTER XVIII
Healthy Spine- Assured Longevity

As we know that life is fast and full of anxieties, it does not elapse without affecting everybody's health. This, of course, brings about some diseases in people. One of such diseases is osteochondrosis. The term "osteochondrosis" is derived from the Latin language, which means degeneration (deterioration and loss of function in the cells of a tissue or organ) caused by dystrophy (a disorder in which an organ or tissue of the body wastes away). This disease is chronic and can lead to an increase in disability among the population. Scientists claim that osteochondrosis causes 17.2% of cases of peripheral nerve diseases which lead to disability. In human, osteochondrosis is not only a genetic disorder but also a consequence of certain diseases as complications during a life-long activity. The human vertebral column is a perfect mechanism. It is extremely flexible, movable and resistant.

The function of internal organs and all sensory organs depends on this spine. Osteochondrosis can cause the diseases of these organs or, conversely, the diseases of these organs can cause osteochondrosis. This part of the torso is created as a chain and consists of approximately 33 bones called vertebrae, which are separated by ligaments and cartilages (intervertebral discs). In an orthostatic (standing) position, this chain is always on clamping regime and it stays in the same position all day when we run or sit.

Intervertebral discs are the most fragile part of the structure, which cannot tolerate unnatural tension, they considerably fine and get injured, often corrupted. As a result, the spinal bones get closer to each other and with their herniations they compress nerves which go from the spine to the internal organs. The blood and lymphatic vessels passed from here are also damaged. Consequently, pain occurs, joints and organs are injured. From the time of adolescence, it is said that the spine starts to encounter some changes. The column can be divided into five different regions, with each region characterized by a different vertebral structure, namely cervical (this region supports the head and it is made up of 7 bones), thoracic (it supports the ribs and made up of 12 bones), lumbar (this region is located in the lower back and is made up of 5 bones), sacral (it is made up of 5 bones) and coccygeal (it is made up of 4-5 bones) vertebrae.

By joining them, the spinal canal is formed, through which the spinal cord passes and 31 pairs of nerve roots spot from that spinal cord. The saddle-shaped nerve which is the largest nerve in the body is accented to be formed in the plexus of lumbar and sacral tufts. Cervical, thoracic, lumbar and sacral radiculitis (osteochondrosis) are differentiated depending on which root is damaged.

Intervertebral discs consist of an outer fibrous ring, the annulus fibrosus disci intervertebralis, which surrounds an inner gel-like center, the nucleus pulposus. The fibrous intervertebral disc contains the nucleus pulposus and this helps to distribute pressure evenly across the disc. Discs, like the hydraulic device, allow vertebrae to move closer to each other and move away from each other. Due to various injurious effects-cum-the effects of exchange, immune, vascular, hormonal and genetic factors, the disc fails.

According to scientists, at first nucleus pulposus changes, and then it leads to its dehydration and withering.

Particularly, if fibrous ring loses its elasticity as a result of physical tension and sudden or prolonged weight falls, cracks and rips may occur, henceforth, chronically dystrophic calcification is observed to appear that is called osteochondrosis. They say that salt is collected. There are three types of different curvatures in the spine such as scoliosis (abnormal lateral curvature), lordosis (excessive inward curvature) and kyphosis (excessive outward curvature). These are considered to be the changes of normal vertebral form. Scoliosis may be congenital (due to the development of abnormal vertebrae) but more commonly occurs among children aged 5 to 15 years, especially among students. Under the circumstances of children's uneven sitting at the desk at school, their weight on the spine and muscles does not fall equally. Then the muscles may languish. When children have rachitis (rickets) in childhood and the elderly always carry kinds of stuff with one hand, it also leads to scoliosis. The waist lordosis can be caused by fat accumulation in the abdomen, which can deform the spine.

The affected part of the spinal column is difficult and painful to move. Treatment of gymnastics and massage are administered by the doctor in case of lordosis.

In cervical osteochondrosis a severe pain may occur, then a person cannot move his neck and his hands become numb at night. When working, his hands quickly feel fatigue. As a result of the distortion of metabolism in the glenohumeral joint (the shoulder joint), movements border and it hurts severely. Osteochondrosis of the shoulder can lead to a chronic and acute deficiency of blood supply to the brain.

In lumbar and sacral osteochondrosis, basically, waist pains, and pain spreads to the back of the foot. Apart from the torment of pain, the skin's sensitivity decreases, the waist & legs become sour and numb as if an ant is clambering. If a patient is not timely cured of the disease, it turns into chronic view. If he gets cold and nervous, does heavy work, coughs, sneezes, walks, sits, stands and physically drees, the pains in the waist and legs escalate.

The vertebra protects the spinal cord in the spinal canal from crushing, stretching and keeps the torso stand-up. It participates as the aegis back wall in forming the thoracic, abdominal and pelvic cavity.

The spinal diseases include congenital defects, the union of more than 2 or 3 vertebrae, extra-vertebrae, etc., and the acquired diseases include spine deformities (curvature, spondylitis) and others.

If somebody listens to the advice on this subject, it will avail certainly:

1. In order to prevent all different defects of the spine, from childhood it is necessary to teach the children to

keep their body aright and to maintain doing complex exercises which strengthens the muscles every day.

2.   It is important to attract the children to work hard, to raise their load, to pay attention to the principles through their youthful attitudes, it is significantly important to teach them to correctly sit at the desk school-aged adolescents should be supervised by school doctors and take steps to remedy static changes on time.

3.   Whoever slowly jogs for only 10-15 minutes every day or once every two days, at least once every three days and then touches the ground in front of his feet with his palms several times without bending his knees, this person's spine, waist & legs will always be healthy.

4. Like all bones, the spine also needs to be fed and cared. It should be fed (anointing) in the summer with little or many oint-

ments (vitamin D) such as aloe vera or soy.

5.   If the spine is damaged (osteochondrosis, neuritis, etc.) and it should be treated by slowly administering 8-10% of an alcoholic solution of Mumijo to painful place for 5-6 minutes within 15-20 days, and also 0,2-0,5 grams of it is consumed per day by mixing milk and honey in 1: 20 ratio.

6.   Do not forget that getting sick in youth with rachitis is mostly caused by working by bending the torso for a long time (such as at the desk, with tools, etc.) which results in postural kyphosis to appear in the thoracic region of the vertebra.

7.   To prevent from scoliosis, children should be taught to properly sit on the desk, to studiously do physical exercises prescribed by the physician, to correctly organize massaging, playing active games, walking outdoors, and for adults, it is important to correctly organize work with rest and engage in production gymnastics while working.

8.   Orthopedist heals the spinal curvature. In order to prevent it, you have to lie on the flat or harder place putting harder pillow while sleeping, do the exercises in the morning and before going to bed, correctly sit on the school desk, at the table, and in the workplace.

9.   Keep away from draft and cold. Keep the waist from overheating, especially try not to have a hot bath. Because of heat effect, spinal muscles may languish.

10.   If you stand for a long time, have some rest. Do not walk for more than 1-2 hours in heel-pieces shoes.

11. At any place (at work or at home), periodically change the maximal position of the waist. Move your arms & legs every 10-15 minutes and occasionally bend yourself back to lie.12.

Do not lie sideways for a long time and fold your head firmly. When lying on the bed, never read and watch TV, it can disorder the blood supply to the brain.

13.   Do not carry heavy loads, especially, with one hand. Always lift loads by bending your legs instead of the waist.

14.   It is inadvisable to do aerobics, shaping, yoga gymnastics and other exercises without a doctor's advice.

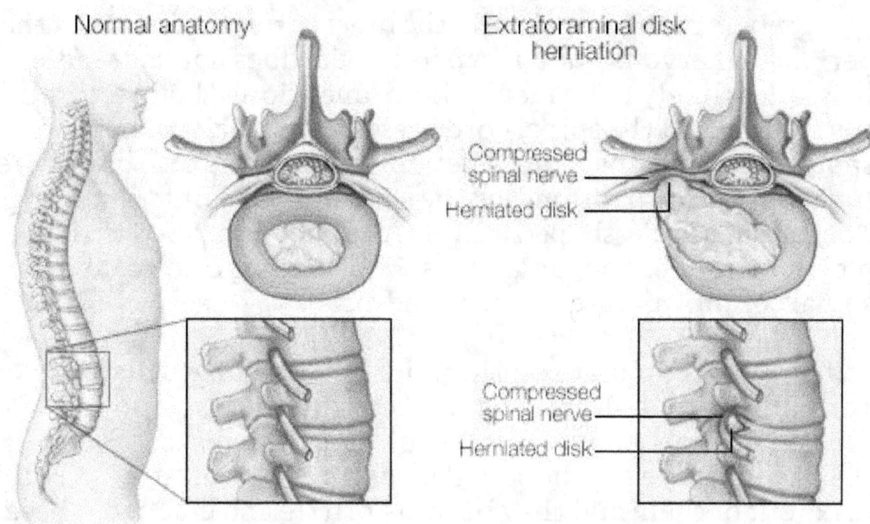

Normal anatomy
Extraforaminal disk herniation
Compressed spinal nerve
Herniated disk
Compressed spinal nerve
Herniated disk

CHAPTER XIX

If You don't wanna Back Pain,...

Radiculitis is an inflammation of nerve roots and their fibers of the spinal cord, the most common disease of the peripheral nervous system. A person who does not have radiculitis is less likely to be met in life. As mentioned before, through the spinal canal the spinal cord passes and 31 pairs of nerve roots spot from that spinal cord. They come out of the thin bony holes in the spinal canal, providing the skin, muscle, joints, and bones. The largest saddle-shaped nerve of the body is formed in the plexus of lumbar and sacral tufts. Radiculitis is often caused by spinal column disease (osteochondrosis).

When salt accumulates at the point where changed discs of vertebrae united, abnormal bony outgrowths (osteophytes) are formed. In most people, slipped discs are the result of wear and tear. Over the years, the spinal discs lose their elasticity. Fluid leaks out of them and they become brittle and cracked. These changes are a normal part of aging, and already start happening when we are young. But not everyone's spinal discs age at the same pace. Very rarely, an accident or severe injury might also cause damage to a spinal disc and leave it herniated.

Spinal discs act as shock absorbers between the vertebrae in our spine. If a spinal disc is no longer able to bear the strain, it can result in a slipped disk. The associated pain probably arises when part of the spinal disc pushes against a nerve in the spinal cord. When herniated disc tissue irritates a nerve root in the region of the lumbar spine, it often causes typical sciatic pain. The nerves that run through the spinal canal connect to the sciatic nerve at the pelvis. The sciatic nerve then runs down the legs. As well as being painful, an irritated sciatic nerve can also cause pins and needles and numbness.

Depending on which nerve root is damaged, radiculitis is divided into different types: cervical radiculitis, thoracic radiculitis, and lumbar-cum-sacral radiculitis. The most common cause of lower back pain is sacral radiculitis.

Herein, the pain occurs in the waist and sacrum, and it also deteriorates when the spine moves. Back pain has been the focus of attention for centuries. The doctors and physicians have taken action to cure this illness. Famous physician, Avicenna points out the causes of lower back pain as follows: waist pains to the patient as a consequence of cold, raw phlegm, excessive fatigue, multiple sexual intercourses, weakness in kidneys, pulmonary edema, and strangulation of the uterus.

At present, lower back pain is not only in adults and the elderly but also in young people. We know that we spend most of our lives in an orthostatic (standing) position. When we stand upright, when we lift the load, when we do labor, jump or even work while we sit, a bigger weight falls on the waist. The lumbar vertebra obtains diseases faster than other vertebrae (various infections, inflammation, poisoning by way of smoking or alcohol, lifting heavy loads, physical tension, injury, and other adverse events affect the cervical & lumbar region of vertebrae and injure it).

Lower back pain is a commonplace for people who work while sitting or standing in the damp place, who have angina often and for the elderly. Spine disorders can also occur in infants, the breastfed babies, and pre-school children.

Scholars claim that this is predominantly caused by the case that the fetus's bone in the womb is not well developed or because of various birth defects. Cervical vertebrae of a baby may be injured during vaginal delivery. In order not to injure a baby, the pregnant woman should be under the supervision of the dispenser, and the doctors should be highly skilled in childbearing. Pregnant women should walk more in the fresh air, do proper nutrition and prevent the fetus from becoming too large. It is absolutely incorrect for women to wear trousers and other tight clothes during pregnancy. The baby should be well developed in the womb and it is significantly important to healthily raise, properly care for and educate the baby after birth.

Helpful tips for back pains are recommended below:

1. If you don't wanna back pain, you should not sit in a cold and damp place, do not make sharp or inaccurate movements, keep your waist from the wind when it sweats, and do not suddenly lift heavy loads.

2. If waist pains to you, immediately go to a doctor (neuropathist, manual therapist).

3. You should not consume meaty, salty and bitter foods. Never become accustomed to harmful habits (alcohol, smoking, etc.).

4. When you have back pain, lie down. According to the doctor's recommendation, it is advisable to take a painkiller and anti-inflammatory medications and to apply mustard plasters, massage, hot baths. If back pain becomes chronic, treatments in resorts and sanatoriums should be done timely.

5. Always try to keep the body upright, if you stay or sit down for a long time, of course, have some rest later.

6. If you work regularly in a sedentary lifestyle, get up every 1 hour, occasionally pull yourself back and lie down.

7. Physical education and sport are practical in preventing back pains.

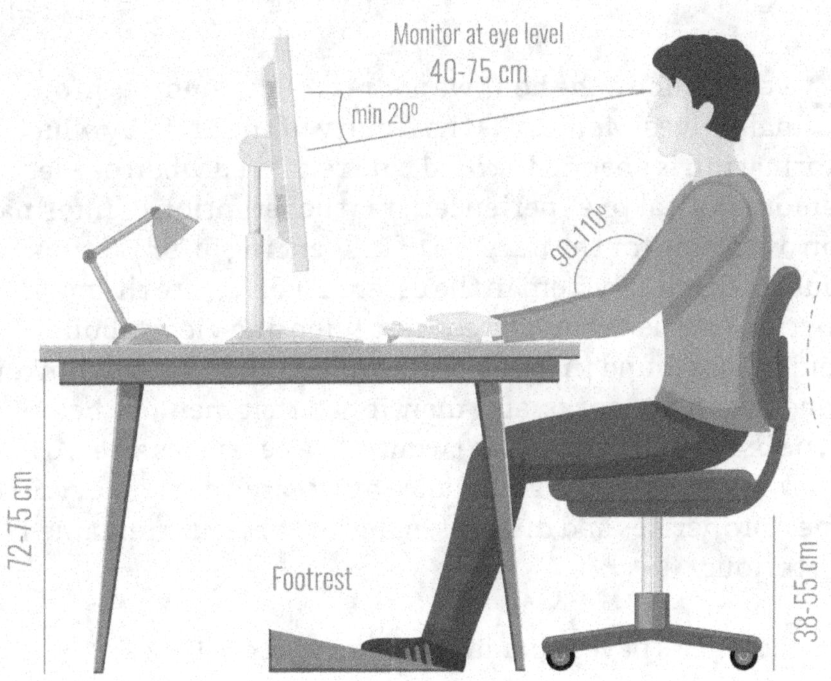

Monitor at eye level
40-75 cm
min 20º
90-110º
72-75 cm
Footrest
38-55 cm

CHAPTER XX
Progressive Memory Loss

"Memory loss or cognitive distortion often results from cold and humidity, sometimes from cerebral edemas, especially cold edemas."

(Avicenna)

Every hour on the hour we address our memories in our daily lives. Memory is the faculty of the brain by which information is encoded, stored, and retrieved when needed. Memory is vital to experiences, it is the retention of information over time for the purpose of influencing future action. Nous and limbic system in the cerebral cortex are the main functions of the brain. The earliest scientific views about memory are found in Greek philosophers and Eastern thinkers. Avicenna, in his works, also mentioned that memory belongs to the brain function. In the twenty-five centuries after Aristotle's era, despite the abundance of research on memory, its types, properties and diseases, many of the issues remained mysterious.

Psychologists have separated memory into 4 types:

1. Memorization and performance of actions;

2. Memorization of images, which is divided into various parts such as seeing, hearing, sensory memory, etc.;

3. Logical memory, which is about memorizing, knowing and repeating the thoughts, ideas, and mental conclusions. This kind of memory is directly linked to education.

4. Emotional memory (sensation, mental experience),

which is about memorizing and repeating feelings with objects which have created them.

Although human memory and its possibilities are the most extensively studied fields in psychology, they are still accented to be fully uncovered. Human beings cannot imagine what happens without memories but know that they cannot be the supreme beings, in general, without memories. In some children, the birth aptitudes are very early detected. There are congenital talented children who have been enrolled in the Institute by their 12-13 years old at 3-4 grades. As psychologist N. Leites points out that when a child unremittingly strives for knowledge and mental work from younger ages, his abilities will well develop. The wunderkinder are smarter enough than their ages.

We know a lot of wunderkinder in the history of world culture. For example, Victor Hugo was rewarded and honored by the French Academy of Sciences at the age of 15. Mozart reached to write more than one hundred plays at the age of 6 and wrote his first opera at age 12. Bolonia's Philharmonic academy elected 14-years-old Mozart as an academician since he was a very gifted and cerebral person. Abdullah Qadiri finished writing his novel called "Bygone Days" during his adolescence. Griboyedov, Metchnikoff, and others were also wunderkinder in their youth. But as the child grows, the pace of his development may change.

We are convinced that there is always a constant proportion between the depth of the memory and the talent of a person.

There are many examples of that. Here are some of them: the astronomer Ulugh Beg Mirza very ably kept his own compiled schedules in his memory. One day he had to recompile the lost schedule. Then, when compared to the original one after it was found, the figures were matched almost exactly. Or, just have a look at Muhammad al-Bukhari, only one example of the power of his memory suffices: one day, the scholars told Bukhari 40 hadiths by changing them designedly to test his memory and asked him how the correct should be. By then Muhammad al-Bukhari had memorized each hadith said by other scholars in the wrong way. When the word turned to him, he looked at each of them, the first thing he mentioned was the incorrect variant, then the correct one, videlicet "You said so, but the actual one is like this". Only then all these scholars capitulated to Muhammad al-Bukhari and his knowledge. It is well known from the history that Ali-Shir Nava'i had memorized the works of his teachers at the age of

6.   When his father took the book out of his hand, he began to tell them by memory.

The famous composer Sergei Rachmaninoff memorized the composed music for a fortepiano that he once heard, and after a while, he could play the music easily.

The memory of world champion Alexander Alekhine was unique. He kept all the chess parties he had played in his memory.

One of the renowned physicists of the twentieth century, Enrico Fermi, had never forgotten the words in the book which he wrote it once and did not ever retake it for his whole life. As far as the human brain is concerned, according to scientists, it can store 8 decimal sign, 7 composite letters, 4-5 numbers, 5 synonyms and meaningful words in a limitedly simultaneous way. However, in life, there were some well-known people who had weakened memory. For instance, Walter Scott, in his old age, was amazed when people read his poems to him and then asked, "Who is the author of this great works?". The novelist, Dostoevsky, forgot the names of even the main heroes of his novel called "Crime and Punishment". "Botanists' father", Carl Linnaeus, even dreamed of his own works by saying "What good books!? I wish I could have written them". There are many people who have

strong memories around us. We often admire that they can re-
tain stories and facts for a long time. But we forget that we also
have these opportunities. For this, we can expand the abilities of
our memories by training them.

It is well known that if the child, along with the development of
his brain in the uterus of his mother, grows healthy and properly
educated after childbirth and, especially, has a liberal attitude
with the outside world, he is highly likely to grow on with the
great nous and have a growth mindset. For a child to become
intelligent, he should be properly educated from the day of his
birth, of course, some of the deficiencies can be precluded during the period of growth.

Memory is a collection of information stored throughout the
brain as groups of neurons, which is gradually amassed since
childhood. The information learned and retained throughout
the lifetime is preserved in the brain and becomes our invis-
ible golden source. As the child's brain is well-developed, he is
highly likely to be curious to know about the surroundings, his
memory will be eidetic. Information reaches through the eyes,
ears, skin, and sensory organs to the brain. Whenever a child or
adult is rich in information, the knowledge base broadens.

Memory is closely interconnected with functions such as peak-
ing, reading, computing, and thinking which are dependent on
the superior activity of the cerebral cortex and the accumulation
of those functions are emphasized to be mind and memory.

Therefore, in order to rescue memory from changes, declines
or degradations, one has to beware of that the single part or
point of the brain should be undamaged or uninjured.

Scientists believe that a correlation between human memory
and aging is enormously relative. For example, Alzheimer's is
a brain disease that causes a slow decline in memory, thinking

and reasoning skills or we will cause this decline, that is, with old age, we will be physically weak and are less likely to use our brain. This leads to sloth of the brain, absentmindedness, and finally memory loss. The power required by physical labor does not require the use of memory. According to Frangistan researchers, one of the main reasons for the degradation of the human brain and its capacity is laziness, escape from a cognitive activity. Yes, literally, laziness of cognitive activity can first lead to absentmindedness, and then to the deterioration of memory.

Absentmindedness is a psychiatric disorder, that is, an instability of attention, being distracted, the premier signs of which are inattentiveness, neglectfulness, and indolence in working. The negligence during placing something somewhere can catalyze failure to find something needed, even when searching with inattentiveness.

In psychiatry, hypomnesia (impaired memory), amnesia (loss of memory due usually to brain injury, shock, fatigue, repression, or illness), or hypermnesia (abnormally vivid or complete memory or recall of the past) can be observed. In some disorders, memory is severely destructed: the events that never happened to the patient seem to have been experienced, in other words, confabulation (memory error defined as the production of fabricated, distorted, or misinterpreted memories about oneself or the world, without the conscious intention to deceive) or a patient thinks that what has once happened appears to have happened today or yesterday that is called pseudoreminiscence (an error of memory consisting in an illusory recall of an experience that one has not had). These false memories are caused by serious mental illnesses.

These disorders are caused by and include cerebral atherosclerosis, intracerebral hemorrhage, physical injury, severe poisoning (eg, Korsakoff psychosis, which is a late complication of persistent Wernicke encephalopathy and results in memory deficits, confusion, and behavioral changes. Korsakoff psychosis occurs in 80% of untreated patients with Wernicke encephalopathy; severe alcoholism is a common underlying condition. Along with memory impairment, a polyneuritis is seen to befall) and so forth. The memory disorder can be terminated by treating the fundamental disease. In alcoholics and chain-smokers who are under the influence of alcohol, cigarette, naswar, and others, the neurons are rapidly eroded, and as we grow older, their number declines, thereby they will be insufficient to manage the body's activity, and they die prematurely.

Alcohol, tobacco, and naswar also reduce the life expectancy, not just because of its toxic effect on the body, but also it makes a person insane, lose memory and causes a decline in critical thinking. In fact, drinking and smoking can bring about harm not only to one's self but to those around them.

The cerebral cortex has more than 14 billion neurons and hundred thousand billion intercellular connections that determine the mental & spiritual world and capacity of human being. Scientists believe that the brain can instantly analyze the information it receives with its incredible speed and draw conclusions.

Thus, memory belongs to the superior function of the brain, which develops during the person's lifetime and according to the capacity and nervous system stability. Usually, as we grow older, our mentalities also increase. Suppose that we unthinkingly did something wrong in our youth, and now we try to fix that by comparing or contrasting it with dissimilar events, it works like this.

Here are some helpful tips on this subject:

1. As stated above, memory belongs to the superior function

of the brain, due to this, it is important to properly care, develop and bring up as well as keep from injury, trauma, and nervousness starting from the periods of pregnancy and infancy.

2.   We need to protect the cells of the nervous system, which serve our memory without asking for gratitude, from various internal and external influences because of the fact that the nerve cells cannot be restored.

3.   Never make your memory busy with daily & miscellaneously paltry and tricky details. Desultory people are considered to be absentminded.

4.   Keep in mind that odors (flowers, herbs, and trees) are the best means to reinstate your memory vividly & vitally.

5.   When atmospheric pressure is high, people think accurately & evidently, and when atmospheric pressure drops, their memory deteriorates.

6.   Using sleeping pills and consuming foods poor in protein, vitamins, calcium, magnesium and glutamic acid can lower recollection

7. Do not forget that daily smoking decreases cognition by 4.42%, observation by 7.09%, a speed of movement by 1,02% and memorization by 5.55%.

8.   Normal usage of tea, coffee, infusion & decoctions of medicinal herbs improves the brain function and the memory capacity. Synthetic medicines should only be used with a doctor's permission.

9.   In order to find out if you have an observation, listening, or a tendency of writing & drawing, just take three small texts, read

the first one inside you, let someone read the other to you, and write down the third one. Then you will determine which text steeps deeper into your memory.

10. Memorizing poems & proses, and monologues, painting, carving, crafting, dressmaking, knitting, assembling a puzzle, playing musical instruments (such as guitar, piano, etc.) are the best methods to exercise memory.

11. To improve memory, consume beet, carrot, cabbage, pumpkin, banana, fig, pineapple, apple, lemon, orange, persimmon, berries, strawberries, raspberries, dried apricot, legumes, nuts, honey, egg, dairy products, fish, and lamb & mutton.

12. It benefits the blood of those who are absentminded if the one tablespoon of haw infusion is often consumed half an hour before eating.

13. Follow the right lifestyle (eating, working, resting, sleeping, exercising, doing sports). Avoid harmful habits (drinking, smoking, etc.). Then consciousness, intelligence, mind, and memory are highly likely to be powerful and advanced.

Alzheimer's disease brain comparison

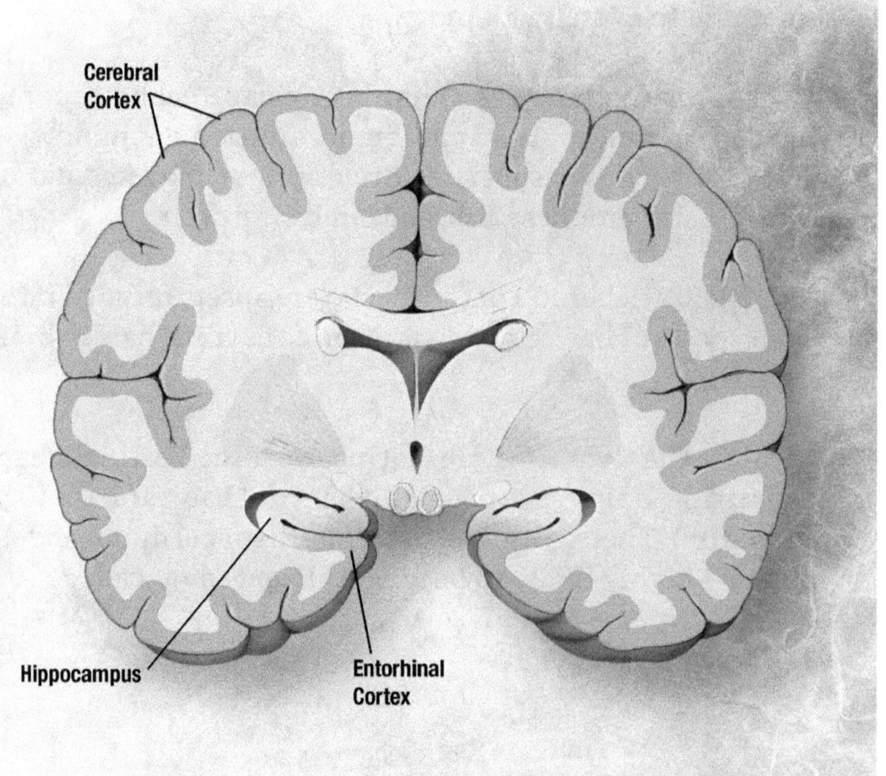

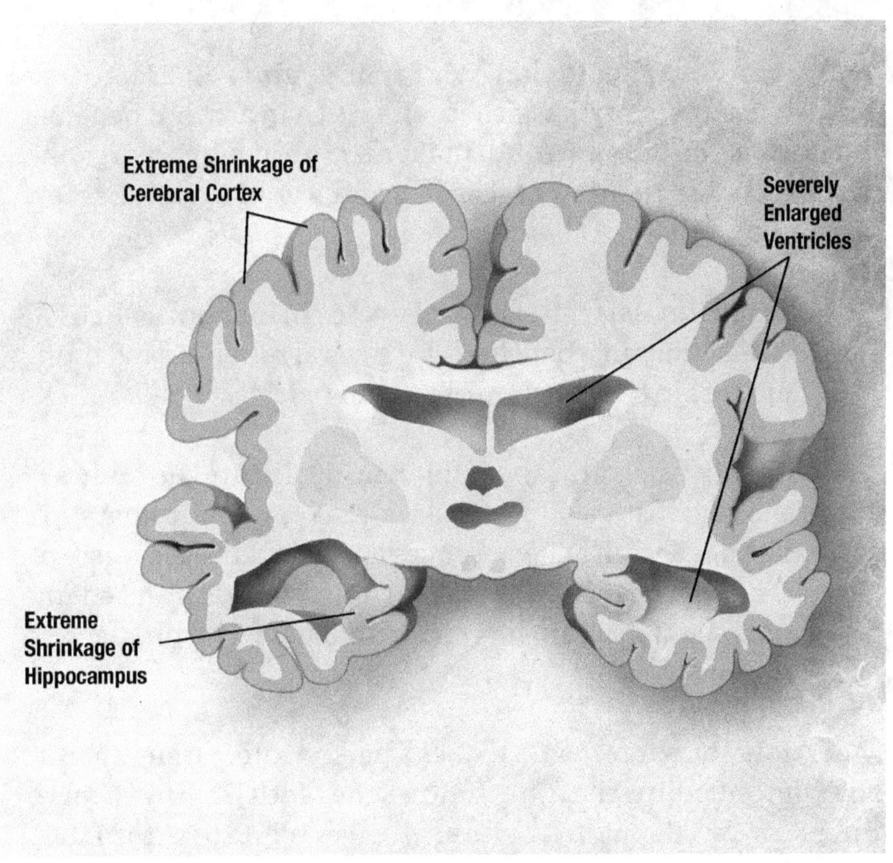
Extreme Shrinkage of
Cerebral Cortex
Severely
Enlarged
Ventricles
Extreme
Shrinkage of
Hippocampus

CHAPTER XXI

Narcomania-
Life-Threatening Disease

The famous theologian, Ibn Taymiyyah, says: "Narcotics are worse off in terms of their effects than alcohol because it destroys the human mind, makes the vital human organs (such as their hands & feet) inactive for a while and takes it to paralysis".

Theologian Ibn Hajar al-Haytami writes in his book called "Al-Fatawa al-Islamiyah" that there are several religious and mundane damages in the consumption of narcotics.

Narcomania frustrates the human mind, limits the body's endurance against various diseases, makes memory harsh, obsesses the head with ache, exposes the heart disease, disrupts the balance of the mind, gives rise to tuberculosis and edema, disappears shame, generosity and human relationships, and so on.

Additionally, narcomania makes a person idle, careless about the family, bedims the eyes, yellows the teeth leading them to prematurely fall out. In the forenamed book, 120 sorts of the harm that narcomania can inflict people and society are enumerated. In recent years, narcomania has sprouted among women, mainly, young people and that has been bothering the world's healthcare workers. In point of fact, narcomania is a pathological craving for narcotics or alcohol, in other quarters, an uncontrollable desire for narcotics.

Narcotics mainly affect the central nervous system, cause deep changes in the body and lead a person to a crisis. The disease progresses slowly and continues chronically.

Narcotics initially stimulate the sense of joy, amusement, and composure. Usually, narcotists' mood is changeable, their memory and capacity go down, metabolism is disordered, and the function of internal organs change.

According to physicians, deeply mental and physical changes occur as a result of narcotics, includingly, if mental changes such as harshness, mood disorders, memory decline occur in narcotists, then subsequent physical changes such as sweating, heart attack, xerostomia (dry mouth), weight loss, shivering, color fracture, and dilated pupil can happen.

Narcomania originates from a wide variety of narcotics, viz. 369, morphine, cocaine, heroin, and marijuana. The body of those who use these substances gets used to them. Their interest in life ebbs and they gradually focus on narcotics and the ways how to find them. If narcomaniac does not receive timely narcotic, severe mental and physical changes occur in the body.

Experts say that drug addicts have fatuous and annoying mannerism, they cannot desist and become sensitive to different colors and voices. In short, both smoking and narcomania inflict severe consequences. Anyone who thinks about his health and the health of his future children will never touch this perdition of life.

In our country, human health, upbringing the younger generation as healthy, strong and spiritually mature individual is an important issue. Everyone in the community should care about their health by themselves, parents, doctors, and others. That is, the health of a person depends primarily on him.

Doctors say that when the disease progresses, the body's frazzle becomes even more intense now that the potency of narcotic overloads the body, that is, an amount of the previous usage starts to effect badly. A drug addict goes into any mischief to have the next pleasure, does not slip treachery, racketeering, theft, and even murder.

According to scientists, using narcotics negatively affects the body's organs as follows:

1. It affects the nervous system, causing various diseases. For example, refractive errors of vision, a decrease in memory, chronic-psychiatric and nervous-somatic diseases. In dope fiends' family, invalid and mentally weak children are born.

2. Young people's enthusiasm to attend educational institutions, classes, and prepare for the lesson will be greatly reduced. As a result, the desire to study and learn a profession & craft disappears.

3.The smoke of hashish has a negative effect on the digestive organs by passing through the oral cavity, the white enamel of the teeth becomes yellowed, its strength is lost, cracks appear in the crown, and appetite decreases.

4. The fetid smell always comes from the body of dope fiends. Their color is low, the skin color becomes a yellowish & murky, sore marks overrun the skin, and hair quickly drops.

5. The findings indicate that 15 percent of the physical disabilities observed in men are directly related to narcomania.

6. It also negatively affects the normal course of pregnancy. In other words, the toxic substances go into the blood of the fetus in the womb. As a result, a fetal heart rate increases.

Female narcotists have slow placental blood circulation, which in turn causes oxygen deficiency in the fetal body's tissues. Therefore, they often encounter many varied problems such as preeclampsia which may lead to placental abruption, fetal distress, respiratory distress in the newborn, and uterine rupture are uncommon complications of labor, various defects in the fetal growth & development and so on.

7. Women who use narcotics lose their shame, their sexual desire increases. The color of the body also yellows, skin loses softness and rapidly wrinkle, voice becomes provocative, they have frequent headaches, breath is pressed, pains appear around the heart, and arterial pressure rises.

8. Narcotics have a detrimental effect on vision nerve. The narcotist's eyes redden and the sharpness of vision becomes blunt. If a person smokes hashish chronically, when he is old, an iris behind the cornea of the eye disappears, and blurriness draws the eyes, and his eyes become fatigued when he reads.

We got acquainted with the terrible consequences of Narcomania. But it is easier to prevent it than treating drug addicts. If someone is snagged by the halter of narcomania and cannot snatch away from it, he/she should immediately go to the appropriate treatment facilities.

It will be all right if we preclude Narcomania from being sprouted, and those who have been accustomed to this harmful habit should be timely identified and timely treated.

Long-term effects of
Heroin

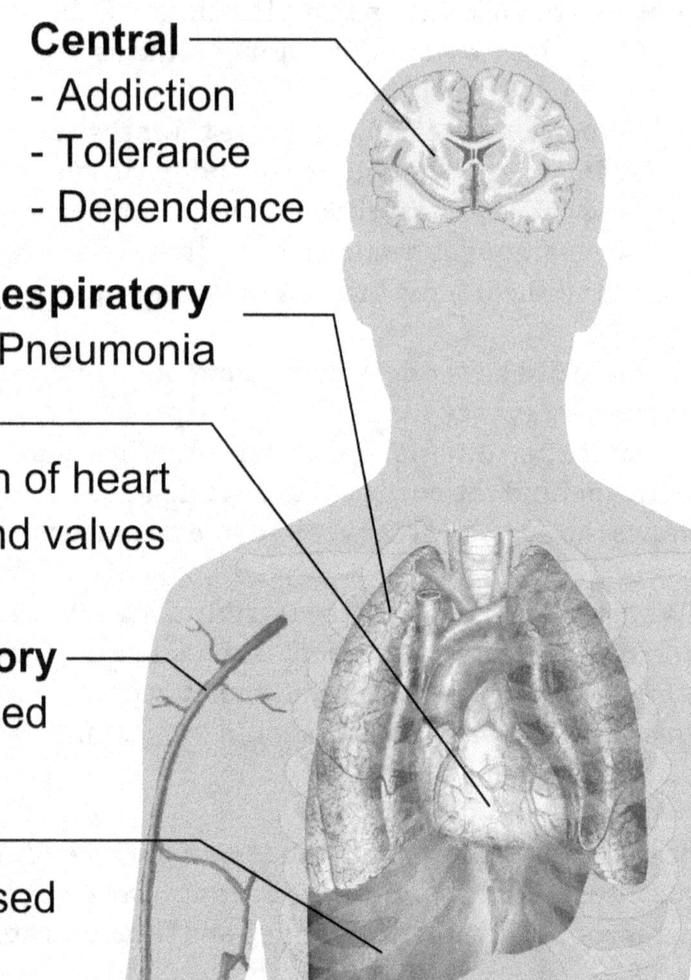

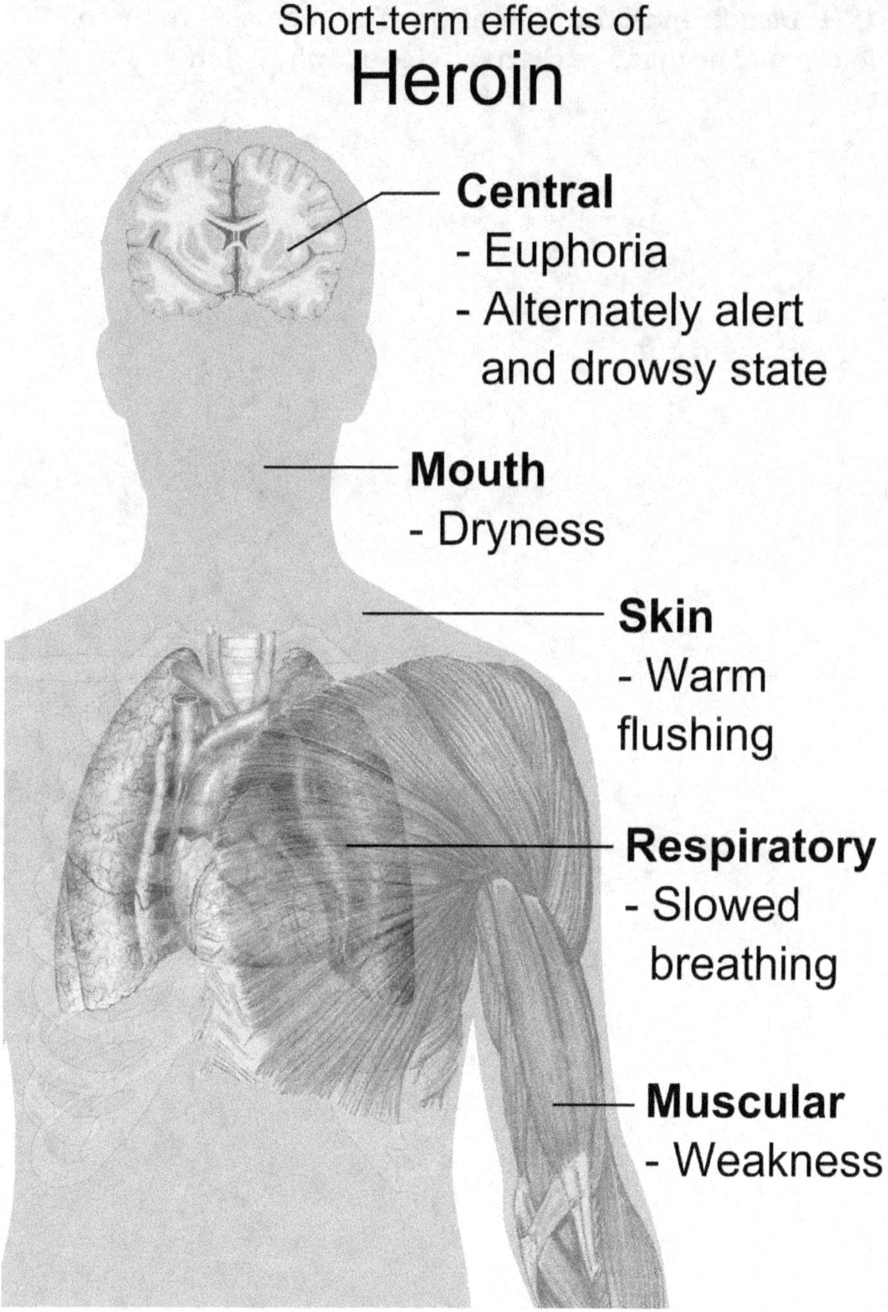

Short-term effects of
Heroin
Central
- Euphoria
- Alternately alert and drowsy state
Mouth
- Dryness
Skin
- Warm flushing
Respiratory
- Slowed breathing
Muscular
- Weakness

NOTE: Dear friends, the utilization of medicinal herbs in this book should be made with the advice of a physician.

CHAPTER XXII

Which is the Best way of Living Life?

Before answering this question I want to just
ask a   question.

So just open your eyes, look within and answer it honestly!

Are you satisfied with the life you're living?

Our attitude is never to be satisfied, never enough, never. No one is ever satisfied. And without satisfaction living life in the best way is impossible.

So be satisfied with whatever you have.

Further coming to the main question the best way of living life is to follow these simple and most important rules of life but without satisfaction all this are worthless.

1. ENVY is a WASTE of TIME. You already have all you need or definitely will get what you really, really want.

2. Do not TAKE yourself too Seriously. NO ONE else does.

3. LIVE with the 3 E's: ENERGY, ENTHUSIASM, EMPATHY.

4. DREAM more while you are AWAKE.

5. PLAY more GAMES.

6. DRINK plenty of WATER. "Drink at least 2 Litres of water per day."

7. SLEEP for 8 HOURS a day.

8. Eat more FOODS that grow on TREES & PLANTS and eat less food that is manufactured in plants.

9. Make TIME to practice MEDITATION, YOGA & PRAYER. Meditation is the KEY to SUCCESS. Trust me!

10. Realize that LIFE is a SCHOOL and you are here to LEARN. Problems are simply part of the Curriculum that appears and fades away like ALGEBRA class but the lessons you learned will last a LIFETIME.

11. Do not have NEGATIVE thoughts or things you cannot control. Instead, invest your ENERGY in the POSITIVE present moment.

12. FORGET issues of the PAST. Do not remind your partner his/her MISTAKES of the past.

13. Do not WASTE your precious energy on GOSSIP.

14. Try to MAKE at least three PEOPLE SMILE each day.

15. READ more BOOKS than you did last month.

16. Spend TIME with PEOPLE over the age of 70 and under the age of 6.

17. However good or bad a SITUATION is, It will CHANGE.

18. Your job won't take CARE of you when you are sick. Your FRIENDS will. STAY in TOUCH.

19. Get rid of anything that is not USE-FUL, BEAUTIFUL or JOYFUL.

20.   You do not have to win every argument. AGREE to DISAGREE.

21. Life is too short to waste time HATING People.
So, get rid of those ILL FEELINGS.

22.   SMILE and LAUGH more.

23.   Take care of eating habits. Eat breakfast like a KING,
lunch like a PRINCE and dinner like a PAUPER.

24.   Make PEACE with your PAST so it won't
spoil the PRESENT.

25.   Sit in SILENCE for at least 10 MINUTES each day.

26.   Take 10-30 MINUTES of JOG every day.

27.   Each day GIVE something GOOD to OTHERS.

28.   Do not overdo. KEEP your LIMITS.

29.   DO NOT COMPARE your LIFE to others'. You have
no idea what their journey is all about.

30.   FORGIVE EVERYONE for everything.

31. TIME HEALS everything.

32.   The BEST is yet to COME.

33.   No matter how you feel, GET UP, DRESS UP and SHOW UP.

34.   ENJOY LIFE each moment, try new things.

35.   CALL your FAMILY often.

36.   Your innermost is always happy. So, BE HAPPY.

37.   No one is in charge of YOUR HAPPINESS except YOU.

38.   What other PEOPLE THINK of you is
NONE of your BUSINESS.

39.   When you awake alive in the morning, THANK GOD for it.

40.   LOVE YOURSELF, because you are UNIQUE
and WONDERFUL in your own way.

I think these are some points which may be helpful to
live life in the best way and happily too.
But remember happiness always lies in satisfaction.
Therefore,

"Enjoy the satisfaction that comes from doing little things well."
(H. Jackson Brown, Jr.)

"Keep a quiet heart,
Sit like a tortoise,
Walk sprightly like a pigeon,
Sleep like a dog."
(Li Ching-Yuen)